JEMMA KIDD
make-up MASTERCLASS

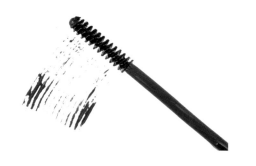

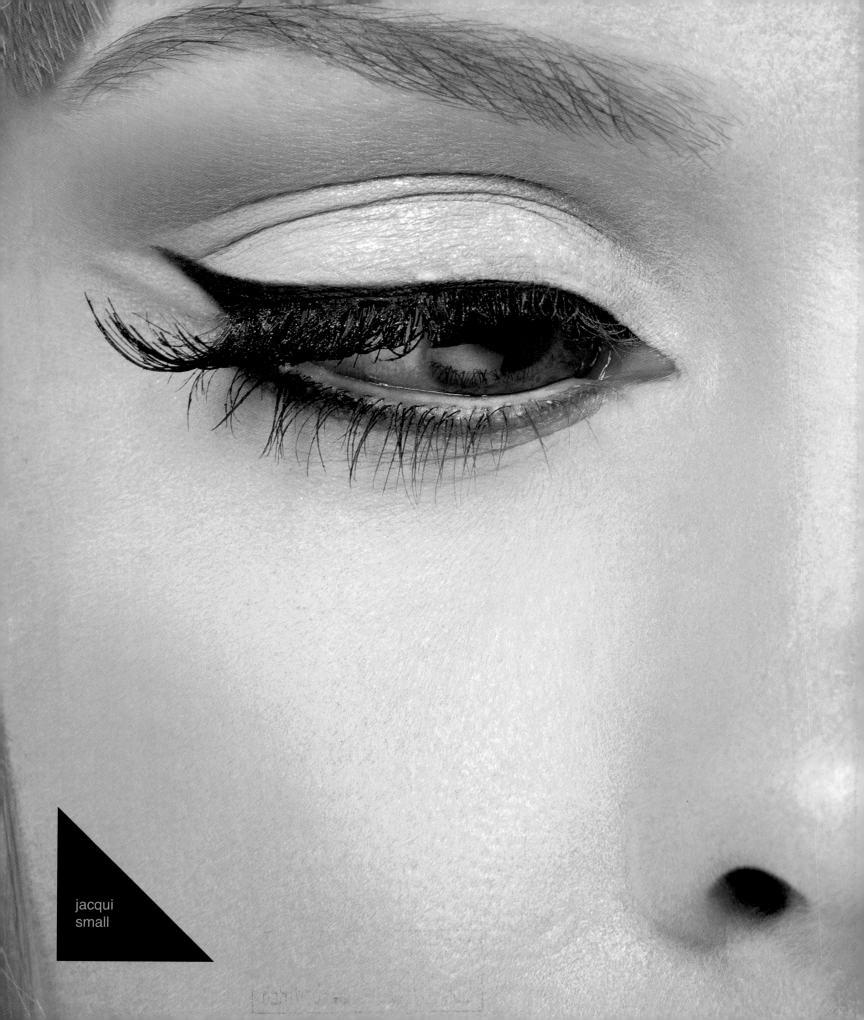

jacqui
small

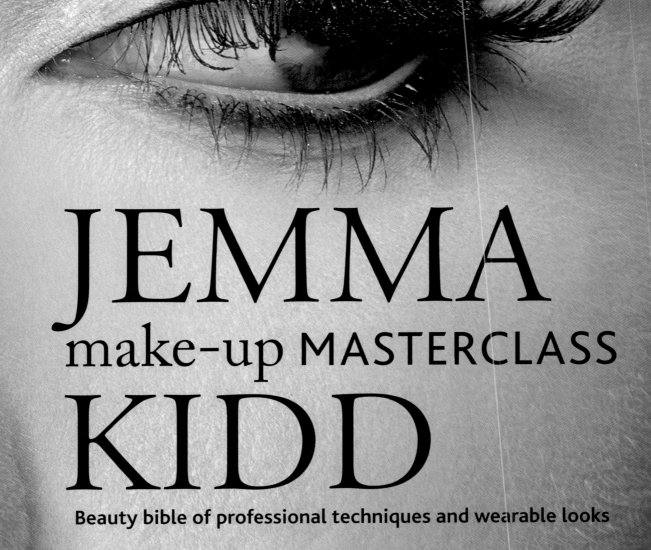

JEMMA
make-up MASTERCLASS
KIDD

Beauty bible of professional techniques and wearable looks

PHOTOGRAPHS BY VIKKI GRANT • TEXT BY ZIA MATTOCKS

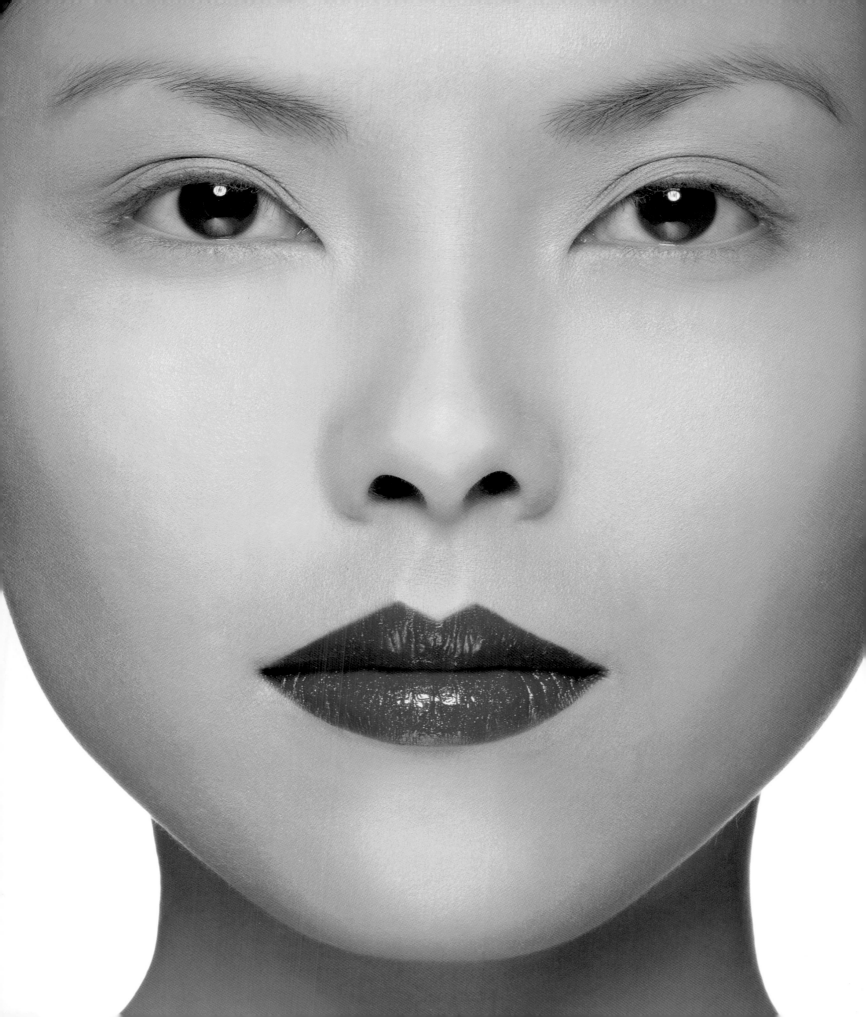

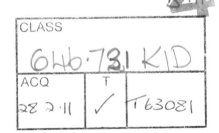

First published in 2009 by Jacqui Small,
7 Greenland Street, London NW1 0ND
Text copyright © Jemma Kidd 2009
Photography, design and layout copyright
© Jacqui Small 2009
The author's moral rights have been asserted.
Publisher Jacqui Small
Editorial Manager Lesley Felce
Commissioning Editor Zia Mattocks
Art Director Lawrence Morton
Production Peter Colley

ISBN 978 1 906417 29 1
A catalogue record for this book is available
from the British Library.
2011 2010
10 9 8 7 6 5 4 3
Printed and bound in Singapore

FOREWORD

This book is the culmination of all that I've learnt during my career as a make-up artist, in particular since founding the Jemma Kidd Make Up School in 2003. It's essentially a distillation of the school's philosophy and the basis of what we teach, which has evolved over the years through working with David Horne, the Education Director, and learning from the women I teach.

When I first learnt to do make-up professionally, I really felt the power of it – how it makes you feel and gives you confidence. When I was travelling the world as a freelance make-up artist, women would often say, 'I'd love to learn how to put make-up on properly – my mother taught me and I've been wearing it the same way ever since.' Whenever I was at home, I'd give make-up lessons to daughters of family friends, and that gave me a far greater sense of achievement than making up models for fashion shoots. As my passion for teaching grew, I realized that there are lots of girls who want to

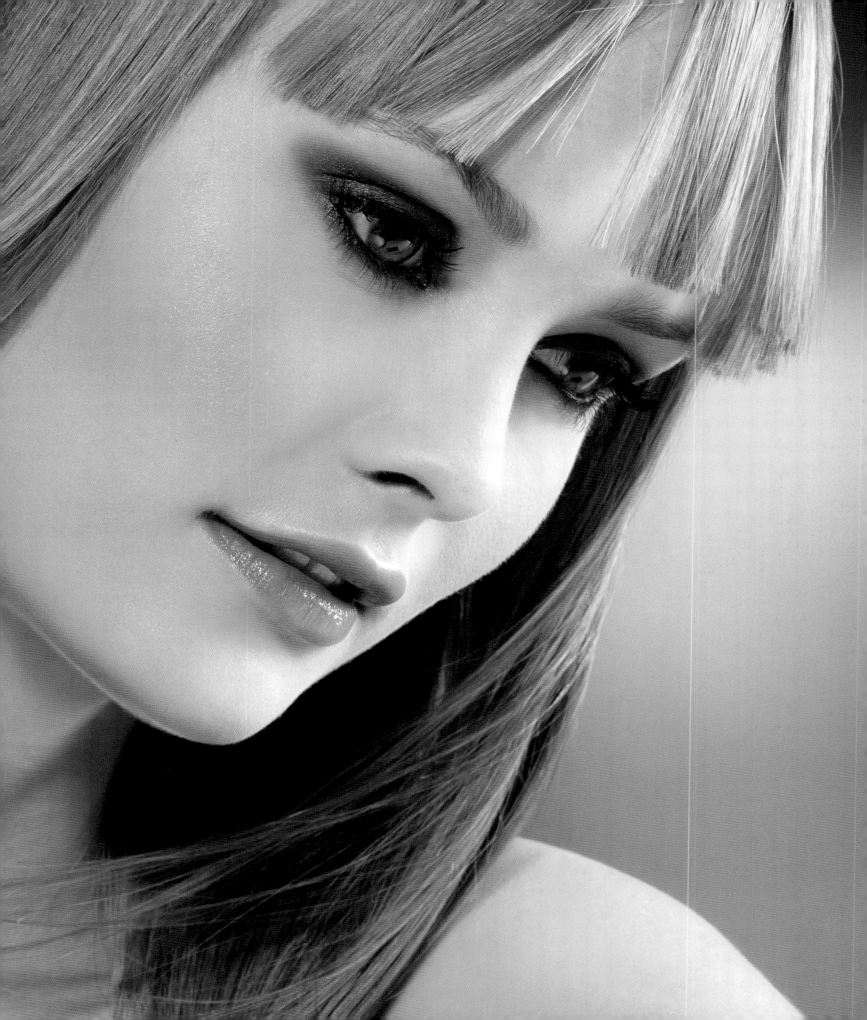

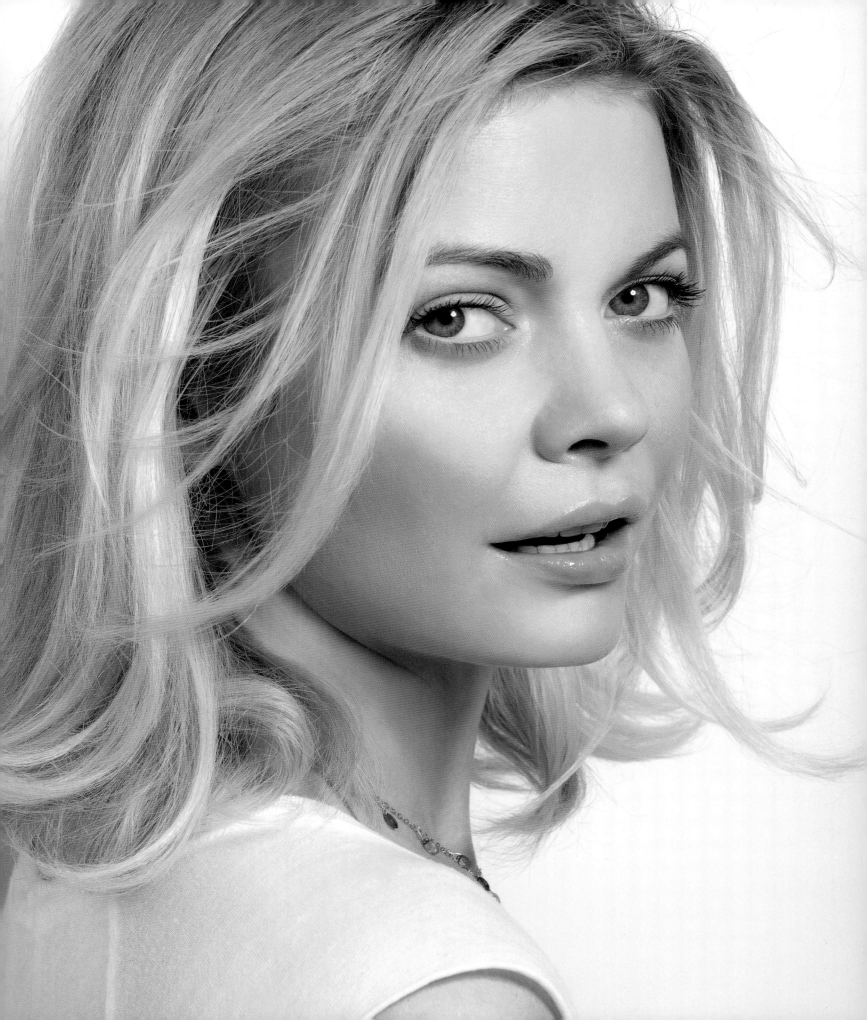

REVEALING BEAUTY

I believe that a woman should view make-up as a powerful tool that can be used to enhance her best features, give her confidence in the way she looks and let her inner beauty shine.

With body image at the forefront of today's media-dominated world, it's no surprise that a woman's perception of how she looks affects how she feels about other aspects of her life. If a woman feels confident about the way she looks, everything seems more rosy and achievable. Many women make the mistake of using make-up as a mask to hide behind, yet once you understand make-up and know how it works, you can easily learn how to bring out the best in your features to reveal your natural beauty.

Make-up shouldn't be intimidating – there are no rules, just guidelines and techniques, so see it as something fun to play around and experiment with until you work out what suits you. It can give you the power to turn a bad day into a good day and change your mood or persona in an instant, taking you from a fresh-faced beauty to a sultry vamp. There are all sorts of tips and tricks that you can learn to make yourself look and feel better – from how to even out your skin tone, to concealing blemishes, to recognizing your eye shape and understanding what works for you.

Practising a good skincare regime is fundamentally important – if you have good skin, you won't need to wear much make-up, which is a joy. You don't need to spend a fortune on expensive products, but do focus on keeping skin moisturized and hydrated, always wear SPF, take your make-up off at night and treat yourself to occasional facials. I'm always on a quest for perfect skin and I've decided that the best things you can do are to eat a healthy diet and drink plenty of water – it's boring, but it makes such a difference. On average the body loses 3–4 litres (5–7 pints) of fluid a day and this needs to be replaced. Hydrated skin looks plumper and more youthful, but if that's not enough to convince you, research has shown that good hydration can reduce the risk of certain cancers, heartburn, arthritis, angina, high blood pressure, migraines and headaches. Urine should be colourless; if it looks yellow, your body is dehydrated.

There's so much pressure on women to stay looking young, and it's my opinion that there's nothing wrong with a little subtle intervention if that's what you need to make you feel better about yourself – that's what life's all about. It only becomes unhealthy when you start to change your appearance. My advice is to research any treatment you're considering very thoroughly, go to a reputable recommended consultant and have a full consultation before you go ahead.

Over the years I've developed three cosmetics lines. The first, Jemma Kidd Make Up School, is about translating professional make-up and techniques into an edited range of essentials that every woman should have. Skincare and colour is combined in one high-tech 'skintelligent' range, with step-by-step instructions making each product supremely user-friendly. Jemma Kidd Pro is a capsule collection of backstage essentials, which I developed with a team of make-up artists. The JK line is where I push design boundaries, taking colours from the catwalk to the sidewalk with my personal interpretation of high-fashion trends.

I'm often asked how I come up with new colours and products. The answer is that I get inspiration from everything – from fashion collections, to holidays, to the people I meet – a recent collection came about from admiring the colourful blooms in a rose garden. My team and I look at the products we have and talk about what we'd like to bring out, then we work with a lab to bring new products into being. I value feedback from women who come to the school, who tell me what they need, like and don't like. I often ask them to try out new products and colours, but at the end of the day I have to trust my eye to know what colour combinations work and I go with my instinct.

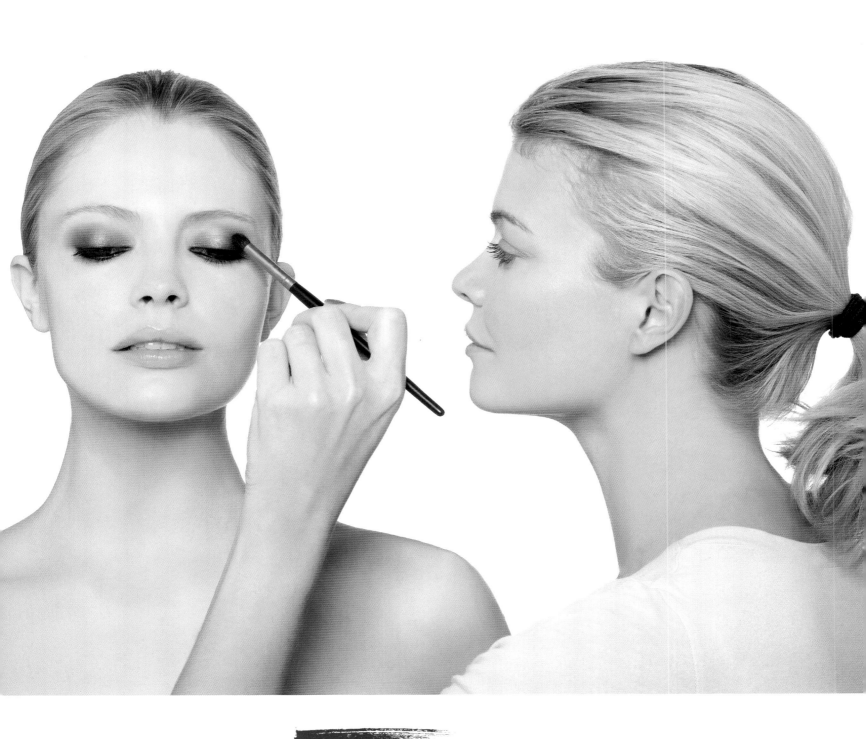

'I love being creative with make-up, but rather than designing high-fashion looks my main goal is to produce beautiful, wearable make-up that makes a woman look like the best version of herself.'

BEHIND THE SCENES

I love the creativity of being a professional make-up artist. If I hadn't followed this path I would probably work in fine art, using paints and canvases instead of make-up and faces to express my love of colour, texture and proportion.

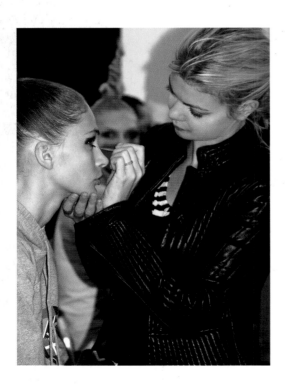

Every face is different, and the key to being a good make-up artist is to be able to interpret face shape and know how to enhance it. You can then have fun creating a look, but you need to be sensitive to the fact that you're dealing with a real person and remember that the aim is to make them feel as good as you think they look. It's not all about you and your creative expression – you need empathy and patience. Some people feel as if you're looking at them naked when you take off their make-up, so you have to be able to gain their trust. It can be an emotional rollercoaster. Doing someone's make-up is a tactile and intimate process, so you tend to bond with your subject quickly.

When you work with a celebrity, your task is to make them look and feel fabulous, so your own ego as an artist has to take a back seat. Celebrities usually have strong ideas about what makes them feel gorgeous and beautiful, so you need to work with them closely to achieve this.

Catwalk shows are all about creating a look and putting on theatre. While you have to be sympathetic if models are tired or run down, essentially they are clothes' horses. The designer is the most important person – it is their look, their story, which everyone else is responsible for interpreting. The designer explains the collection and storyboard, which may be inspired by a film, book, person, place or era. Once you understand the feel of the clothes, you can begin designing the make-up, working closely with the hairstylist. One look has to suit the entire collection, so you have to be careful in your colour choices and take into consideration the time of day the show will be on – make-up needs to be quick to apply if models are likely to be running late from previous shows.

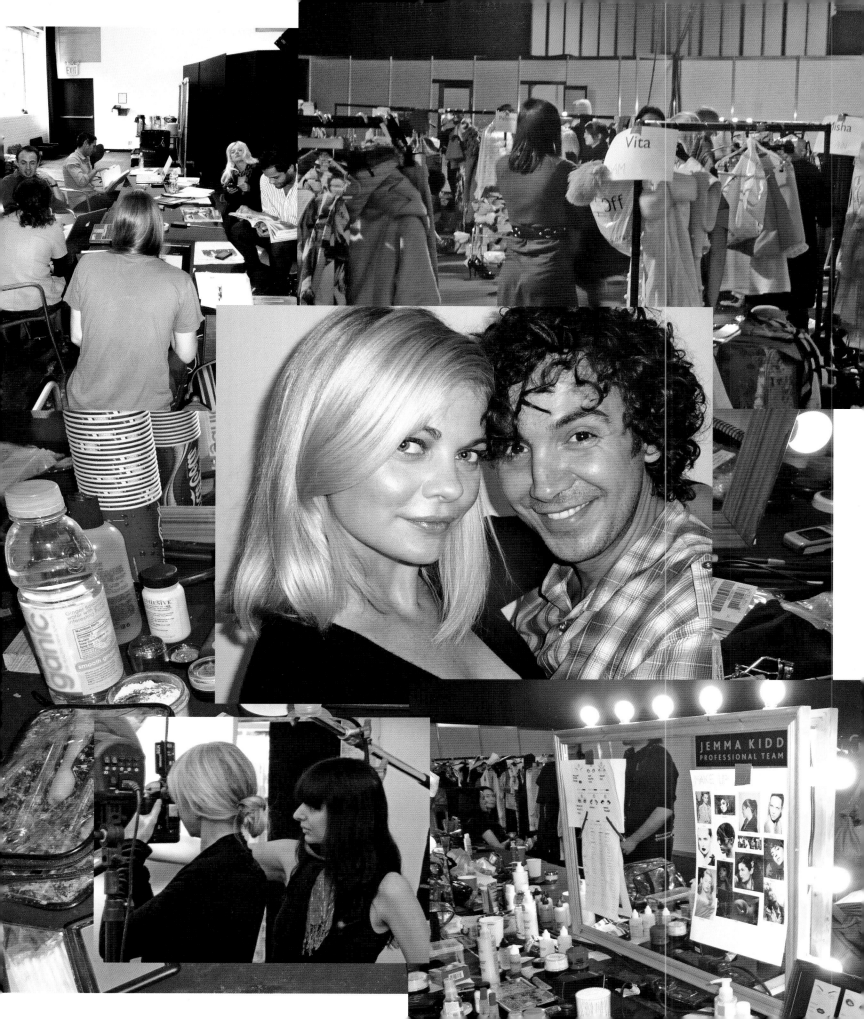

MY ULTIMATE TOP TEN BEAUTY TIPS

1
WELL-GROOMED BROWS FRAME THE FACE. KEEP THEM NEAT AND TIDY AND DEFINE THEM WITH A BROW PENCIL, WORKING FROM THE ARCH OUTWARDS AND THEN ON THE INNER PART IF NEEDED. GO OVER THE SHAPE WITH A BROW POWDER, WHICH WILL SOFTEN THE SHAPE AND MAKE IT LAST LONGER.

2
USE A FLESH-TONED EYELINER ON THE INNER RIM OF THE EYES TO MAKE EYES APPEAR WIDER AND FRESHER AND TO NEUTRALIZE ANY REDNESS. PALE EYELINER INSIDE THE EYE CREATES A MORE OPEN-EYE EFFECT, WHILE DARK EYELINER INSIDE THE EYE CREATES A MORE ELONGATED FOCUS TO THE WIDTH OF THE EYE.

3
HIGHLIGHTER IS A USEFUL TOOL FOR CREATING ILLUSIONS. DAB A CREAMY HIGHLIGHTER UNDERNEATH THE ARCH OF THE BROW TO LIFT THE BROW AND MAKE THE EYES LOOK WIDER. ADD A TOUCH ABOVE THE CUPID'S BOW TO MAKE THE LIPS APPEAR FULLER. YOU CAN ALSO MIX A LITTLE HIGHLIGHTER WITH YOUR FOUNDATION TO GIVE SKIN AN ALL-OVER LUMINOSITY.

4
IF YOU HAVE THIN OR SPARSE EYELASHES, USE AN EYELINER TO FILL IN ANY GAPS BETWEEN THE LASHES AND LIGHTLY DUST THEM WITH POWDER IN BETWEEN COATS OF MASCARA TO ADD VOLUME. IF YOU ARE PRONE TO SMUDGING MASCARA ON YOUR EYELIDS, USE A DROP OF FOUNDATION ON A COTTON BUD TO REMOVE IT.

5
AS WE MATURE, BROWN MASCARA AND EYELINER IS MORE FLATTERING THAN BLACK. GEL AND LIQUID LINERS CAN LOOK HARSH, BUT DAMP EYESHADOW USED AS AN EYELINER WILL FLOW BETTER OVER FINE LINES.

OPT FOR A YELLOW-BASED CONCEALER, AS IT WILL HELP TO CAMOUFLAGE RED OR PURPLE TONES IN BLEMISHES, AND COMPLEMENT ANY SKIN TONE.

IF YOU HAVE DRY SKIN, USE A FOUNDATION AND BLUSH WITH A CRÈME FORMULATION, WHICH WILL HELP TO PLUMP UP THE SKIN AND MAKE IT LOOK SUPER-HYDRATED. FOR MORE MATURE OR TIRED-LOOKING SKIN, TRY MAKE-UP WITH INVIGORATING INGREDIENTS SUCH AS CAFFEINE AND/OR LIGHT-REFLECTING PIGMENTS TO REVITALIZE YOUR LOOK.

IF YOU'RE USING CRÈME BLUSH OR BRONZER, APPLY IT STRAIGHT ON TOP OF LIQUID OR CRÈME FOUNDATION AND BLEND WELL. IF YOU'RE USING POWDER BLUSH OR BRONZER, DUST A FINE LAYER OF TRANSLUCENT POWDER OVER THE FOUNDATION TO SET IT. THIS GIVES A VELVETY FINISH AND THE PERFECT CANVAS FOR APPLYING POWDER BLUSH OR BRONZER – IF YOU APPLY A POWDER FORMULATION DIRECTLY ONTO FOUNDATION, IT WON'T BLEND AND WILL LOOK STREAKY OR PATCHY.

GENTLY BRUSH YOUR LIPS WITH YOUR TOOTHBRUSH AFTER YOU BRUSH YOUR TEETH TO EXFOLIATE THEM AND PREPARE THEM FOR SMOOTH LIPSTICK APPLICATION.

USE LIPLINER ALL OVER THE LIPS, NOT JUST AS AN OUTLINE. THIS WILL GIVE A BETTER FINISH AND WILL HOLD YOUR LIPSTICK FOR LONGER. IF LIPSTICK DOES WEAR OFF, YOU WILL STILL HAVE AN ALL-OVER COLOUR RATHER THAN JUST AN OUTLINE.

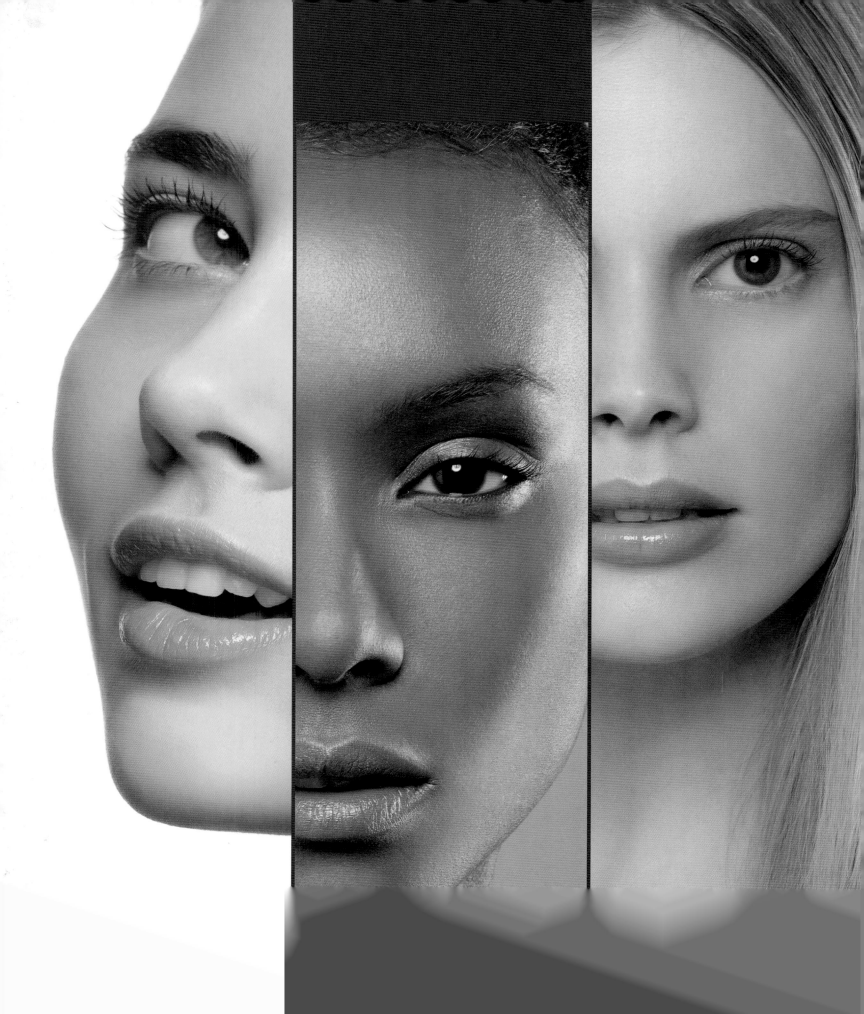

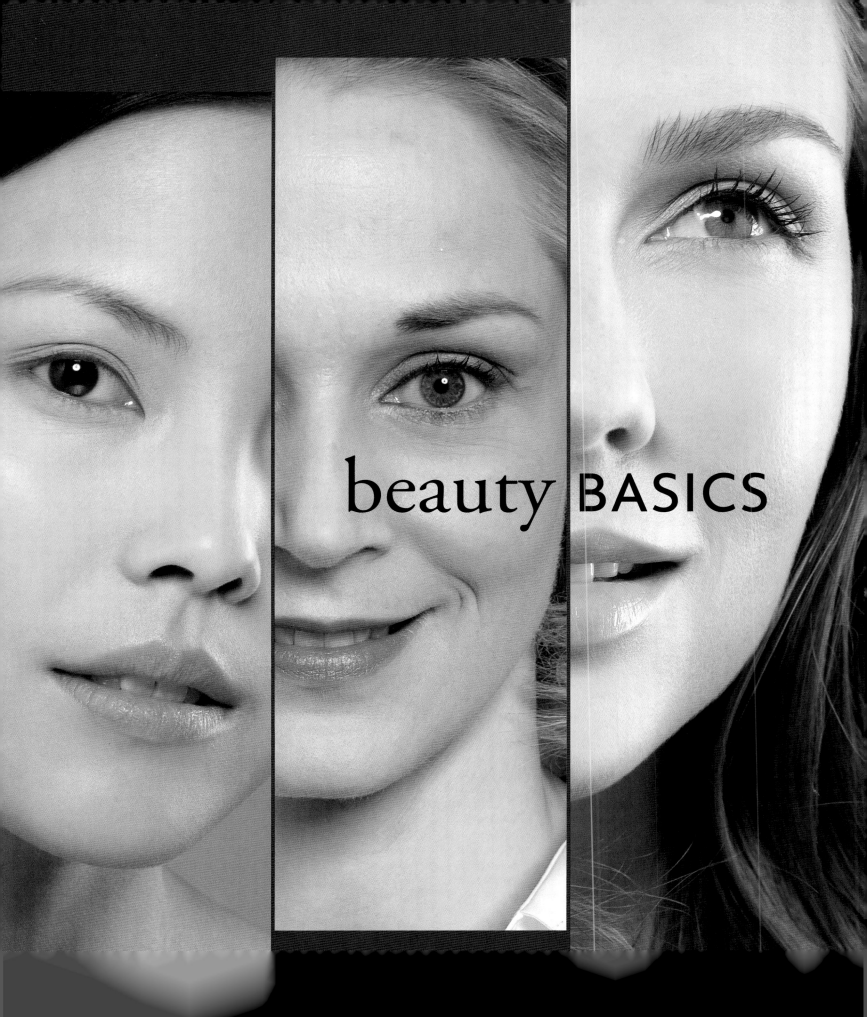

beauty BASICS

SKIN DEEP

The skin is the body's largest organ – if we could shrug it off, its weight would be equivalent to three bags of sugar. It acts as a barrier against the environment and infections, and helps to regulate body temperature and excrete toxins.

Unlike other organs, the skin is visible – a map of your life, complete with freckles, thread veins, open pores, spots, scars and laughter lines. Because it's exposed to the sun, cold, wind and pollutants, the signs of stress will soon show if you don't take care of it. While the condition of the skin is undeniably affected by the external environment, diet, lifestyle, hormonal changes and the passage of time also play a part in its behaviour at any given time.

It is important to be able to recognize your skin's tendencies and characteristics so that you can treat it accordingly and restore balance, but accept that these won't remain constant. Skin may be drier during the winter than the summer, and may be prone to oiliness and breakouts at different times of the month or because of a change of diet or lifestyle. Smoking, too much alcohol and too little sleep can all have a negative impact on the skin's health, making it look dull and dehydrated, while stress can trigger sensitivity and lead to outbreaks of complaints such as eczema and psoriasis.

Normal skin may

» Feel soft and supple with even tone and no enlarged pores..
» Rarely or never suffer from breakouts.
» Never react adversely to skincare products or cosmetics.

Oily skin may

» Look shiny and feel greasy, even after washing.
» Have visible open pores.
» Be prone to breakouts and blackheads.

Sensitive skin may

» Feel itchy or bumpy and look flaky or red.
» Flare up when you use products containing allergens such as fragrance or lanolin.
» Burn easily in the sun.

Dry skin may

» Look flaky and dull and feel tight, especially after washing.
» Show signs of ageing, such as fine lines.
» Have a crepey appearance, especially around the eye area.

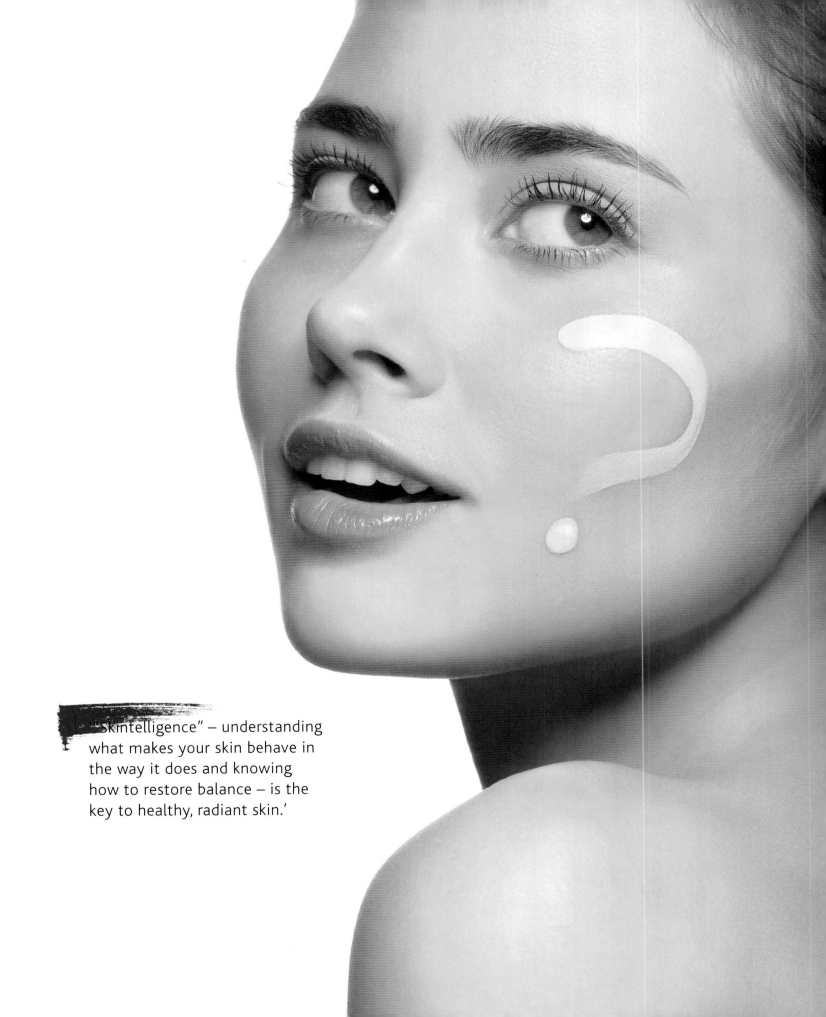

'Skintelligence" – understanding what makes your skin behave in the way it does and knowing how to restore balance – is the key to healthy, radiant skin.'

managing your skin

Normal skin

If you have skin that is neither excessively dry nor oily, nor especially prone to sensitivity, you are lucky enough to have normal skin. Even so, most people's skin goes through phases when it is drier, oilier or more sensitive than at other times. Also termed 'combination' skin by cosmetics companies, normal skin may be slightly dry on the cheeks with greasier patches on and around the nose, chin and forehead, as these areas naturally produce more sebum. No one product can hydrate one area while absorbing oil from another, so the best option is to treat problem areas separately with different products.

The choice of make-up formulations are wider if you have normal skin – anything goes, and it's a matter of trial and error to see what suits you best.

Dry/dehydrated skin

The body loses about 600ml (1 pint) of water a day by evaporation through the skin, and if moisture is lost faster than it can be replaced by underlying tissue, the outer layer becomes dry. Production of sebum, a natural oil, is minimal and pores are almost invisible, so the plus point is that dry skin is less susceptible to breakouts. The downside is that dry skin tends to show signs of ageing and can be flaky.

SOS – how to restore balance

» Drink at least eight glasses of water a day.

» Use skincare products with a high water content.

» Wear a protective moisturizer as a barrier against water loss.

Top make-up tips for dry skin

» Make-up sits on the surface of dry skin, so moisturize well and use an oil serum under foundation.

» A light moisturizing liquid foundation will work better for you than crème or stick formulations.

» Oil-based products glide on easily; powder products sit in creases and draw attention to fine lines and flaky patches.

» Crème blush is preferable to powder blush for the same reason.

My secret Dehydrated skin tends to look worn and lined, whereas skin that is well hydrated looks vibrant and healthy, so investing in the right serums, masks, moisturizers and eye creams is important.

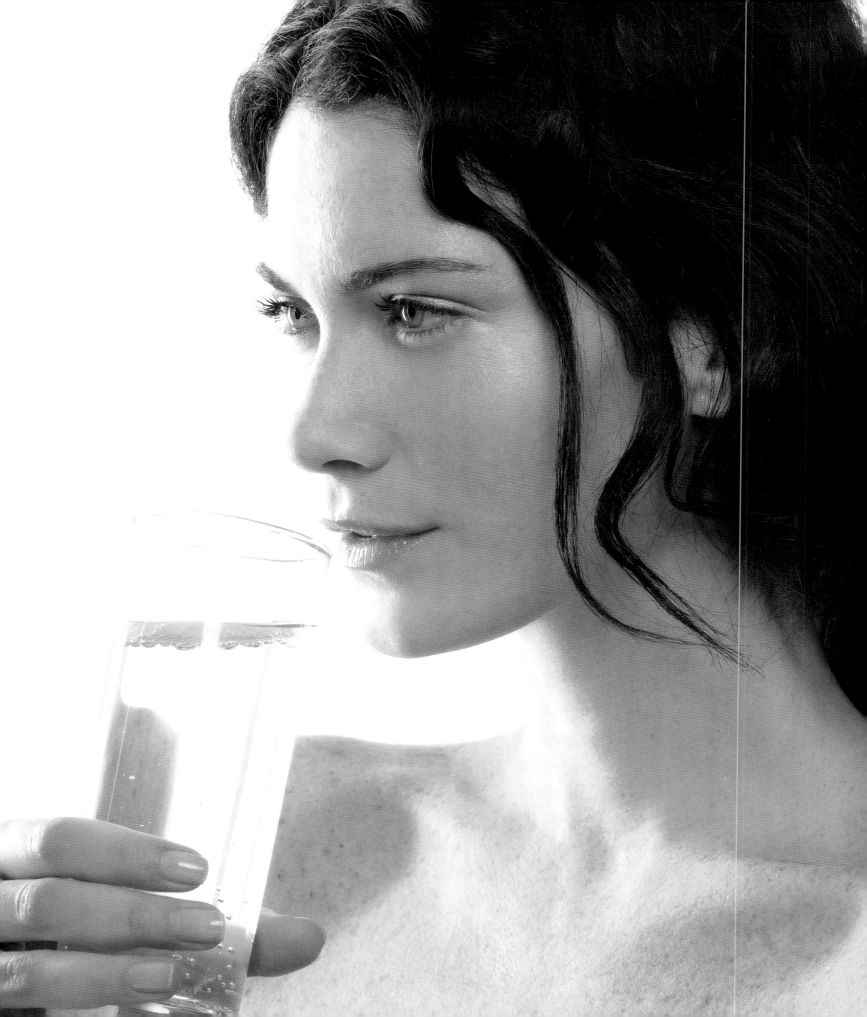

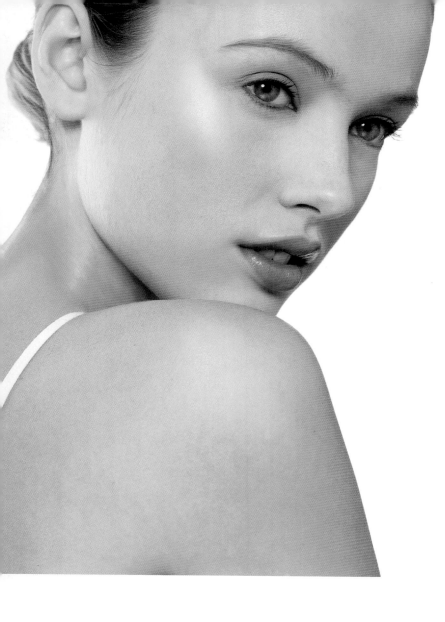

My secret Blotting tissues come in booklets that are easy to carry in your handbag. These are better for quick fixes than powder, which may absorb the oil but will also clog pores and sit on the skin's surface.

Oily skin

Skin produces an oil called sebum, which keeps it supple and healthy and protects it from environmental aggressors. Overactive sebaceous glands result in greasy skin with larger, open pores. It can be more prone to breakouts, as the excess oil blocks the pores and makes the surface shiny, which also makes it harder for some kinds of make-up to stay on (especially on a hot day). On the positive side, women with oily skin tend to have fewer wrinkles.

SOS – how to restore balance

» Keep the skin hydrated as it will try to produce more oil if it feels dry. Use water-based moisturizers or those formulated for oil control.

» Don't overwash the skin, which will stimulate the production of sebum. Use an oil-based cleanser to dissolve excess sebum.

» Avoid oil-stripping products with a high alcohol content. These make the skin feel fresh in the short term, but they are too harsh and will make the problem worse.

Top make-up tips for oily skin

» Use a mattifying primer under foundation to help it to stay on and enable you to use less, reducing the risk of clogged pores and blemishes.

» Silica helps to absorb oil – look for it in primer, foundation and powder. Silica can hold a large amount of oil and keep it locked away from the skin's surface, preventing blocked pores.

» Mineral powder foundations are perfect for very oily skin, as the oil helps the powder to be absorbed, giving a natural finish. Alternatively, use a light foundation and buff your skin with a fine loose powder.

» Avoid crème blushes, bronzers and eyeshadows, which are often wax-based and sit on the skin's surface, leading to blocked pores.

» Oil-free make-up and moisturizers will help to keep you shine-free. Steer clear of products that claim to give a glossy or satin finish, as these contain fats.

Sensitive skin

Some women are allergic to certain ingredients, others have skin so sensitive that any perfume or colouring can make it flare up. Many brands such as Lancôme and Estée Lauder make fragrance-free products, while Origins and Aveda use only organic ingredients. Elave products are affordable and great for sensitive skin (and skin with open pores). Moisturizers with natural ingredients and without perfumes are likely to be more gentle, but be careful because some essential oils and plant extracts can react with the skin. The fewer things there are on the ingredients list, the less likely that the product will react with your skin.

SOS – how to restore balance

» Use hypoallergenic cleansers and moisturizers specially formulated for sensitive skin.

» Avoid harsh products containing alcohol and perfume; instead choose soothing ingredients such as aloe and camomile.

» Don't use harsh exfoliants for cleansing – even rounded beads can overstimulate the skin.

» Investigate organic or natural make-up ranges, but always ask for testers to see how your skin will react before buying.

Top make-up tips for sensitive skin

» Don't wear too much make-up and avoid heavy foundation. Liquid foundation that is silicone-based is less likely to irritate sensitive skin, while hypoallergenic powder formulations contain few preservatives and feel light on the skin.

» If you have a high colour, neutralize the red with concealer or primer before applying any colour to your skin.

» Choose yellow-toned foundation rather than pink. Some companies, such as Prescriptives, can mix foundation specially for you.

» Use a foundation containing sunscreen to keep the amount of product you're wearing to a minimum.

» Try beige or tan colours on your eyes – they cause less irritation to sensitive skin than highly pigmented colours.

» Wax-based pencils tend to cause fewer problems than liquid eyeliners – not least because they are easy to remove.

My secret Wash sponges, brushes and applicators frequently, and throw out old cosmetics. Keeping your products clean is good hygiene in any case, but when you have sensitive skin it's especially important.

problems and solutions

Grown-up acne

Acne should go when you leave your teens, but adults can suffer from breakouts at any age. It is one of the most common problems and can take a lot of effort to get your complexion blemish-free.

Treat it at the salon

» Omnilux Blue uses a spectrally pure blue light source to clear and control acne and kill harmful bacteria. Initially the skin gets worse, but patients can expect to see a 70–80 per cent improvement by the end of the course.

Treat it at home

» Use tea-tree essential oil on a cotton bud to help dry out a breakout.

» Use products that reduce excess oils and keep it clean – Proactiv products are great for acne-prone skin.

» Light-reflecting foundations can show up dents and scars, so choose a perfect colour-match matte foundation.

» Use a medicated concealer that soothes as well as covers – my favourite is by Dr Hauschka.

My secret Those with acne or chickenpox scars may find a primer helpful in smoothing the skin and helping make-up to adhere.

Red cheeks

Skin isn't meant to be one flat colour, but sometimes you may want to tone down redness or spider veins. Broken capillaries can occur for a number of reasons, including UV damage, exposure to extreme weather or even hormonal changes and alcohol.

Treat it at the salon

» Vasculight treatment for thread veins and rosacea is amazing. A laser targets and releases energy in the red pigment of the blood cells, which causes thread veins to close without puncturing them. The body then absorbs the closed vessels over four to eight weeks. Between two and six treatments may be necessary.

Treat it at home

» Use a high-factor sun protection cream (at least SPF 30) every day.

» If skin is well moisturized, you can use a heavier foundation that gives better coverage for red cheeks.

» Use a yellow-toned concealer and pat it on top of foundation on areas of redness or thread veins, then seal with fine powder.

» Use a little highlighter on the tops of the cheekbones and a dusting of bronzer or beige blush to contour. This will make any redness recede.

» Steer clear of bright, candy colours for eyes or lips, as these will bring out the redness in the cheeks. Muted colours will give a more balanced effect.

My secret Red skin on cheeks is often dry, so use a rich moisturizer, such as Dr Hauschka's Rose Cream, to make sure there's no roughness. Clinique also has an anti-redness range. Some skincare specialists claim that natural extracts such as Vitamin K, centella and horse chestnut help to strengthen capillaries and hence reduce broken thread veins.

Scarred, but not for life

When I was little I was bitten by a dog and had a scar on my cheek. For years I was self-conscious about it until I had laser treatment, which helped to reduce it to a thin line.

Treat it at the salon

» Procedures such as laser treatment or topical bleaching gels can be very effective. Different problems have different solutions, so do your homework and meet the specialist for a full consultation.

Treat it at home

» Scars need to be protected from sun and dryness. Use a broad-spectrum high SPF (30+) – Aloe Gator SPF 40+ Gel offers eight hours' protection and is the best I know. Use a gentle cleanser and keep skin well moisturized.

» There are several companies, such as Dermablend, Covermark and Coverblend, which sell concealers and foundations that provide excellent coverage for scars and birthmarks.

» To apply, pat the foundation gently onto the affected area and wait for it to be absorbed, before blending at the edges. Set with powder to prevent any smudges.

My secret Try not to become too self-conscious. Your face is more than a scar and confidence is the key to beauty.

Open pores

Pores can become enlarged through the build-up of grime, excess oil production or simply through ageing. Whatever the cause, they are a magnet for grease and dirt and will ruin your complexion.

Treat it at the salon

» A series of glycolic peels dissolves the top layers of the skin, which reduces the pore size and clears any trapped dirt, shrinking pores.

Treat it at home

» Deep-cleansing masks can draw out impurities and excess oil.

» A splash of cold water or spritz of flower-water toner after cleansing closes pores before applying moisturizer.

» Apply a product that minimizes the appearance of open pores, such as Elave Age Delay Night Treatment or Clinque's Pore Minimizer Instant Perfector gel.

Milia

These are tiny balls of cells that become trapped under the skin and look like little white beads. Eventually they will go by themselves, but there are ways of getting rid of them.

Treat it at the salon

» The Priori Advanced AHA Peel contains lactic acid, which dislodges dead skin cells from the surface of the skin that cover milia, squeezing out the contents and leaving the skin smoother.

Treat it at home

» Try using a self-heating, exfoliating mini-peel treatment.

» Regular exfoliating and a good cleansing regime should keep milia away.

clean up your act

A good skincare routine is the key to healthy, glowing skin. Your twice-daily regime should be to cleanse well and then moisturize. Exfoliate once or twice a week, depending on the product, and use an appropriate treatment mask – deep cleansing, hydrating, nourishing or calming – once or twice a month.

Skin should be spotless before you apply moisturizer or make-up, otherwise pores will become blocked and lead to breakouts. Your face needs to be prepped well to achieve a perfect base – it makes all the difference to the finished result – and at the end of the day, remove all traces of make-up before applying night cream.

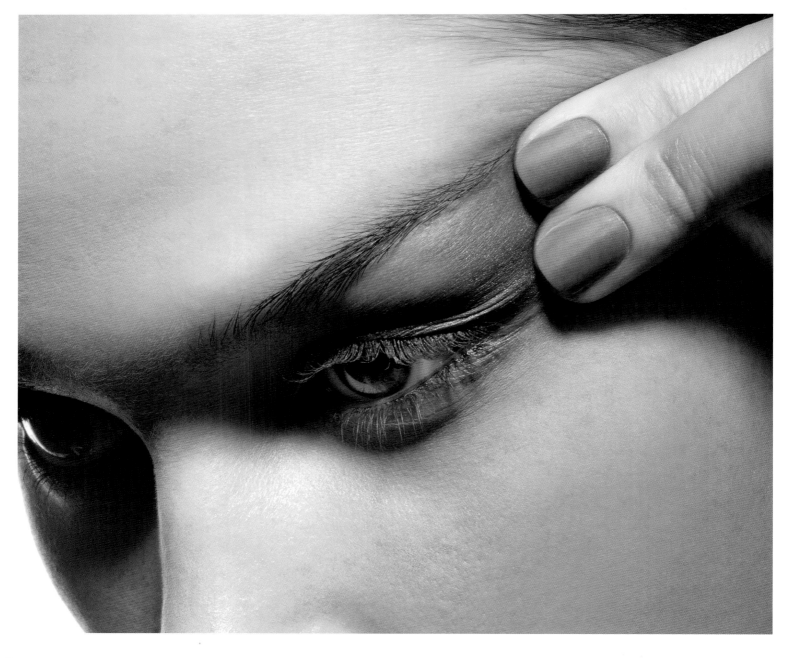

Cleanse

While basic soap and water can upset the pH balance of the skin (soap is alkaline, while the epidermis is acidic) and leave a pore-clogging oily residue, cleansers that you rinse off with water will leave your skin feeling freshest. Try any of the gentle wash-off cleansers available in bars, creams, liquids and foams, which leave skin residue-free without feeling tight and dry. Avoid ingredients such as lanolin or fragrance, which can aggravate the skin, and paraffin and moisturizer, as these may block the pores. Some cleansers come with a muslin cloth that you use to polish and gently exfoliate the skin as you remove the cleanser. You may need a separate eye make-up remover, especially if you use waterproof mascara.

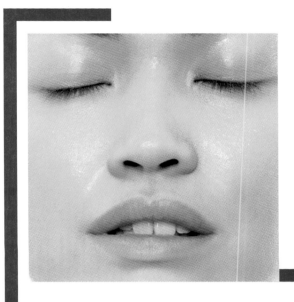

PRE-MAKE-UP ROUTINE

» Cleanse your face and finish with a splash of cold water to close the pores, then gently pat dry.

» Use tweezers to tidy brows and pluck away stray hairs.

» Apply a serum, followed by an appropriate day moisturizer containing SPF 15 or more.

HOME TRUTHS ABOUT CLEANSERS

- Cleanse skin in water at least once a day. Remove stubborn eye make-up with a cream or oil-based cleanser, but afterwards wash the face in warm water using a mild, soap-free cleanser.

- Cleanse thoroughly before putting on a heavier night moisturizer. You must be certain there's no oil or dirt in the pores that will get blocked in and cause blemishes.

- If you come home too tired to cleanse properly, use impregnated wipes. I don't recommend using wipes every day, as they can leave product on the skin and the weave can be harsh on the face.

- Cleanse your neck as well – it is as exposed as your face and is just as likely to show signs of ageing. Use a gentle upward sweeping motion, so as not to pull the skin down.

- For really tough eyeliner or mascara, use a cotton bud dipped in oil-based cleanser to remove product from the roots of the lashes. If you run out of oil cleanser, olive oil works well.

- Use toner only if you have oily or combination skin. If you cleanse with water, normal skin won't require toner. Avoid alcohol-based toners, which strip the skin; instead look for gentle natural flower waters.

Tone

Opinion is divided as to whether a dedicated astringent toner is necessary after cleansing. I believe that if you have normal skin and are using a water-soluble cleanser, a splash of cold water is sufficient to close the pores. If you use an oil or cream cleaner that is not water-soluble, or if you have exceptionally oily skin, toner can help to counteract this, but avoid anything alcohol-based or solutions that contain harsh ingredients such as acids or witch hazel. A light spritz of flower water, such as rose water, can be a great alternative, giving a fresh finish without the unpleasant tightness or drying effect.

Exfoliate

The purpose of exfoliation is to help along a natural process. Skin cells on the surface are essentially dead, and can make the skin feel dry and look dull and lifeless. Exfoliation lifts the dead skin cells away to reveal brighter skin cells beneath.

Skin on the face is delicate, so you should not use a product that is too abrasive. Hot-cloth cleansers are ideal for dry or sensitive skin. They are hydrating and perform gentle exfoliation as you wipe away the product with a muslin cloth (machine-wash the cloth once a week and rinse it between uses to avoid a build-up of bacteria). For normal skin, look for a gentle exfoliant with rounded beads or a micro-dermabrasion technique, and use once or twice a week. Oily skin or skin with blocked pores will benefit from an exfoliator that contains fine granules to slough away dead skin gently.

Moisturize

Get to know your skin so that you can select the right moisturizer. You may decide that you need moisturizer only on certain areas of the face, avoiding oily patches on the nose and chin, for example, or that you need a richer moisturizer in winter to combat the drying effects of cold weather. The skin around the eyes and on the neck is thinner and prone to dryness. Don't forget these areas, as they are often the first to show signs of ageing.

Deeply penetrating facial serums, concentrates and oils can be used on their own or under moisturizer to protect and address skin damage and dehydration. Smooth the product over the face and neck using gentle upward sweeping motions.

TOP TIPS

» When applying thick cream, place a small amount in the palm of your hand and press your hands together to warm it. Cup your face with your hands, firmly pressing the cream into the skin rather than rubbing it.

» Make sure your day cream contains SPF 15 or more to protect your skin from ultraviolet light.

» The area around the eyes is thinner and more sensitive than the rest of the face, so a specially formulated eye cream is essential.

» Use a night cream that stimulates cell regeneration. Skin repairs itself at night and the temperature of the skin increases during sleep, aiding the absorption of active ingredients.

TOP TIP

Exfoliate using very gentle circular motions over the cheeks, forehead, nose and chin, avoiding the delicate area around the eyes.

'Be extremely gentle with your skin – never scrub, rub or tug at it, which could damage and stretch it.'

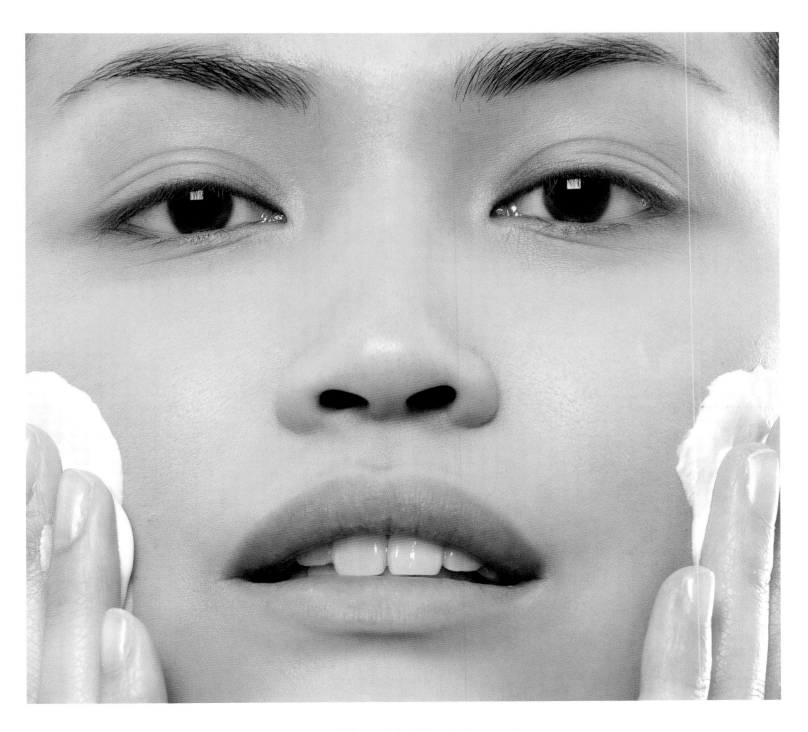

POST-MAKE-UP ROUTINE

» Soak a cotton pad in eye make-up remover and press gently onto the closed eye to dissolve the make-up, then wipe all traces away. Use a cotton bud to remove mascara and eyeliner from the roots of the lashes.

» Cleanse your face and tone with a splash of cold water.

» Apply serum, if required, followed by an appropriate night moisturizer.

sun sense

Whenever you're outside you need protection from both UVA and UVB light – even on a cloudy day, 80 per cent of the sun's UV rays reach the ground. Just walking to work or spending your lunch break outside mean you should be protected, even if you spend the rest of the day in an office. If you are fair-skinned, blonde or a redhead, there is a higher risk of photoageing and skin cancers. There's no need to wear the thick sunscreen you might wear for the beach – think about your skincare regime and decide which combination of products will protect you best.

What to look for

A sun protection factor (SPF) of 15 means that skin can stay in sunlight for 15 times its normal limit – 20 minutes in most cases. SPF 15 is a minimum for the face, but 30 is preferable for fair skin. Make sure the sunscreen contains protection against UVA rays, which are the most damaging in the long term, leading to premature ageing, and UVB rays, which cause sunburn. SPF 15 offers enough protection if you'll be out for a short time, while SPF 30 is appropriate if you'll be outside all day. SPF 15 should be used at all times on anyone aged 18 and under to prevent permanent damage.

Moisturizers

A cream sunscreen can feel heavy, so try a gel or oil-free sunscreen if you have oily skin – apply it a good 10 minutes before make-up to let it soak in. For day-to-day use, choose a moisturizer with SPF 15 that is light enough to wear under make-up without feeling greasy. If you are going to be outside for much of the day, or in a warm climate, use a moisturizer with SPF 30 or higher. Try to find one that contains vitamins A, C and E for added protection.

If your skin is sensitive, choose a hypoallergenic and unfragranced moisturizer or serum. Skin that's been exposed to the sun reacts to perfume, and this is especially true of the undereye area. Most eye creams contain SPF, but I recommend a light, easily absorbed gel for every day.

Make-up

Many foundations contain suncreen, but this isn't sufficient to protect the skin for extended periods in the sun. I recommend applying foundation sparingly, so I would never rely on it alone for sun protection – combine with a lightweight SPF moisturizer or primer. For very sheer coverage, try an oil-free tinted moisturizer with SPF.

In hot weather heavy foundation is a mistake, as it can slide off sunscreen. Mineral foundation could have been made for summer – even those with dry skin will find that this works better in hot weather, but apply it sparingly and work well with a brush to ensure it is properly settled into the skin. Layer it over a moisturizer that contains SPF, especially if your skin is dry.

TOP TIPS

» Don't neglect your décolletage, neck, ears and hands. Apply moisturizer with a minimum of SPF 15 and don't forget to reapply after washing hands.

» Many sunblocks for lips contain petroleum and zinc, which can be drying or give a white finish. Use a lip balm with SPF, or apply a moisturizing balm and layer with a tinted lipstick that contains a high SPF.

» Avoid the midday sun and keep a tube of facial sunscreen in your bag.

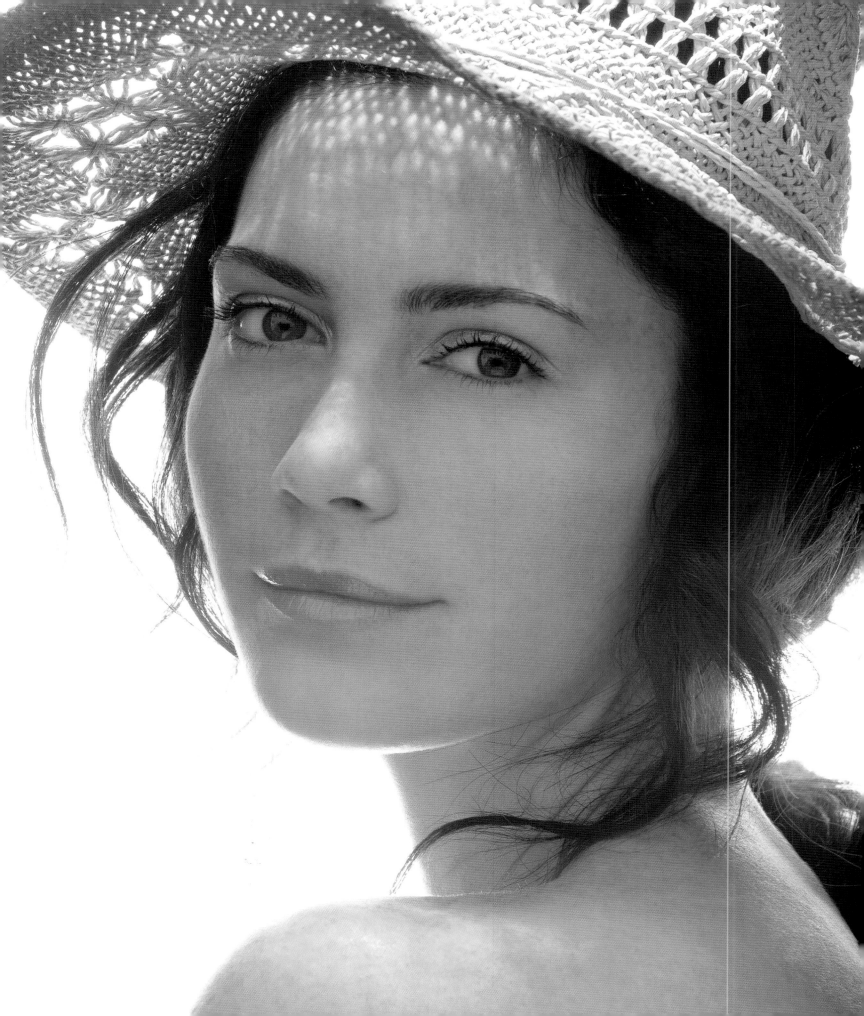

TOP TEN TIPS FOR RADIANT SKIN

ALWAYS WEAR A SUNSCREEN WITH SPF 15 OR HIGHER TO AVOID PREMATURE SKIN DAMAGE DUE TO PHOTOAGEING. THE EASIEST WAY TO DO THIS IS TO USE MOISTURIZER AND FOUNDATION WITH BUILT-IN SPF.

EXFOLIATE REGULARLY TO REMOVE DEAD CELLS AND LEAVE SKIN LOOKING FRESH AND HEALTHY. EITHER USE A GENTLE EXFOLIATING WASH EVERY DAY OR AN EXFOLIATING CREAM TWO TO THREE TIMES PER WEEK. DON'T SCRUB TOO HARD, AS THIS CAN DAMAGE THE CAPILLARIES.

TO KEEP YOUR SKIN LOOKING BEAUTIFUL, EAT PLENTY OF FRESH FRUIT AND VEGETABLES, WHICH ARE HIGH IN ANTIOXIDANTS AND HELP TO PROTECT THE SKIN FROM ENVIRONMENTAL DAMAGE. OMEGA 3-6-9 SUPPLEMENTS ARE RECOMMENDED FOR GOOD SKIN.

REGULAR EXERCISE INCREASES BLOOD CIRCULATION, WHICH CARRIES MORE NUTRIENTS TO THE SKIN AND HELPS WITH THE RENEWAL OF SKIN CELLS.

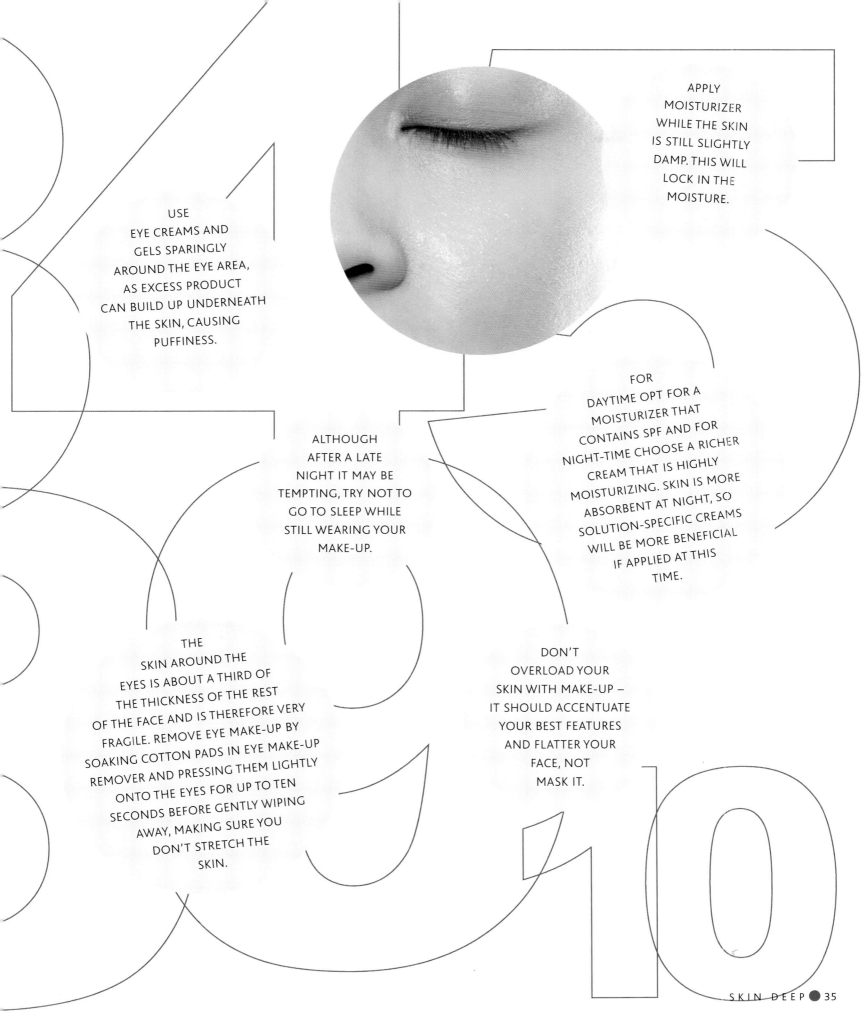

USE EYE CREAMS AND GELS SPARINGLY AROUND THE EYE AREA, AS EXCESS PRODUCT CAN BUILD UP UNDERNEATH THE SKIN, CAUSING PUFFINESS.

APPLY MOISTURIZER WHILE THE SKIN IS STILL SLIGHTLY DAMP. THIS WILL LOCK IN THE MOISTURE.

ALTHOUGH AFTER A LATE NIGHT IT MAY BE TEMPTING, TRY NOT TO GO TO SLEEP WHILE STILL WEARING YOUR MAKE-UP.

FOR DAYTIME OPT FOR A MOISTURIZER THAT CONTAINS SPF AND FOR NIGHT-TIME CHOOSE A RICHER CREAM THAT IS HIGHLY MOISTURIZING. SKIN IS MORE ABSORBENT AT NIGHT, SO SOLUTION-SPECIFIC CREAMS WILL BE MORE BENEFICIAL IF APPLIED AT THIS TIME.

THE SKIN AROUND THE EYES IS ABOUT A THIRD OF THE THICKNESS OF THE REST OF THE FACE AND IS THEREFORE VERY FRAGILE. REMOVE EYE MAKE-UP BY SOAKING COTTON PADS IN EYE MAKE-UP REMOVER AND PRESSING THEM LIGHTLY ONTO THE EYES FOR UP TO TEN SECONDS BEFORE GENTLY WIPING AWAY, MAKING SURE YOU DON'T STRETCH THE SKIN.

DON'T OVERLOAD YOUR SKIN WITH MAKE-UP – IT SHOULD ACCENTUATE YOUR BEST FEATURES AND FLATTER YOUR FACE, NOT MASK IT.

SKIN TONE

Globalization has led to a myriad subtly and dramatically different skin tones being found all over the world – and almost as many different colours and textures of make-up.

'As a rule, skin with pink undertones suits cool blue-based colours, while warmer orange-based shades are more flattering on skin with yellow undertones.'

The sophisticated formulations of modern cosmetics make the majority of today's products far more forgiving and versatile than traditional make-up. In addition, pushing the boundaries by wearing clashing colours and mixed-up textures is often viewed as a fashion-forward statement, rather than a hideous mistake. Yet if you're after a natural, purely beauty-enhancing look, there are certain guidelines to follow.

The science

The colour of skin, hair and eyes is genetic and is governed largely by the quantity of melanin and carotene, pigments that add brown and yellow respectively. Melanin is formed in cells known as melanocytes within membrane-bound bodies called melanosomes. The most common forms of melanin are eumelanin, a brown-black polymer, and pheomelanin, a red-brown polymer largely responsible for red hair and freckles. The various hues and degrees of pigmentation found in skin are related to the number, size and distribution of melanosomes – hence the higher the concentration of eumelanin, the darker the skin will appear, and vice versa. The melanocytes are triggered to produce more melanin as a response to UV damage, which is why skin tans after exposure to the sun.

The other factor that influences skin colour is the visibility of the blood vessels, which adds pink or blue tone. Oxygenated blood is bright red while deoxygenated blood is darker red, which is why skin flushes pink after exercise when oxygenated blood is pumping faster around the body and blood vessels are rising to the surface of the skin to cool the body down. The less pigmentation in the skin (that is, the less melanin), the more visible the blood vessels will be.

PINK   YELLOW

RED   OLIVE

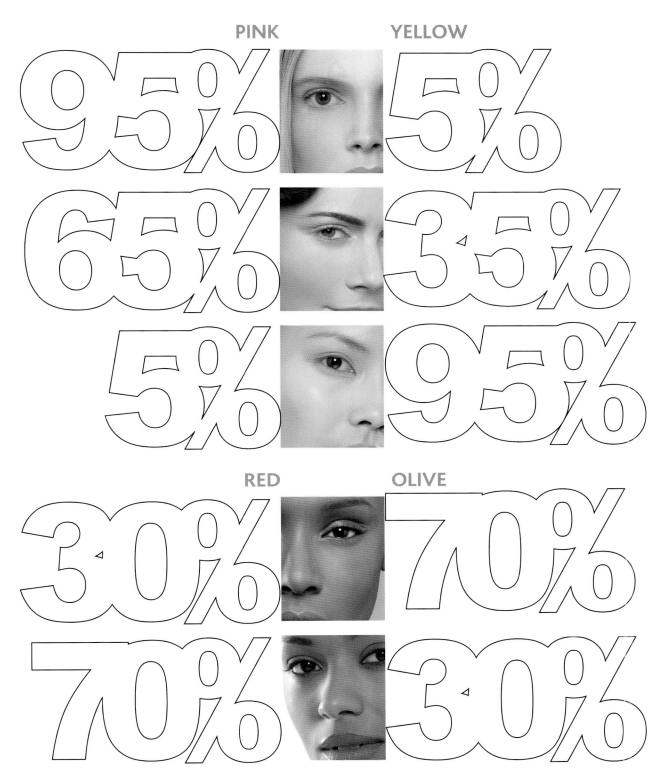

Identify your skin's dominant undertone, which will be either pink or yellow, then decide how light or dark it is.

» Porcelain skin is approximately 95 per cent pink and 5 per cent yellow

» Fair skin is approximately 65 per cent pink and 35 per cent yellow

» Olive skin is approximately 5 per cent pink and 95 per cent yellow

» Deep skin can be either red- or olive-toned.

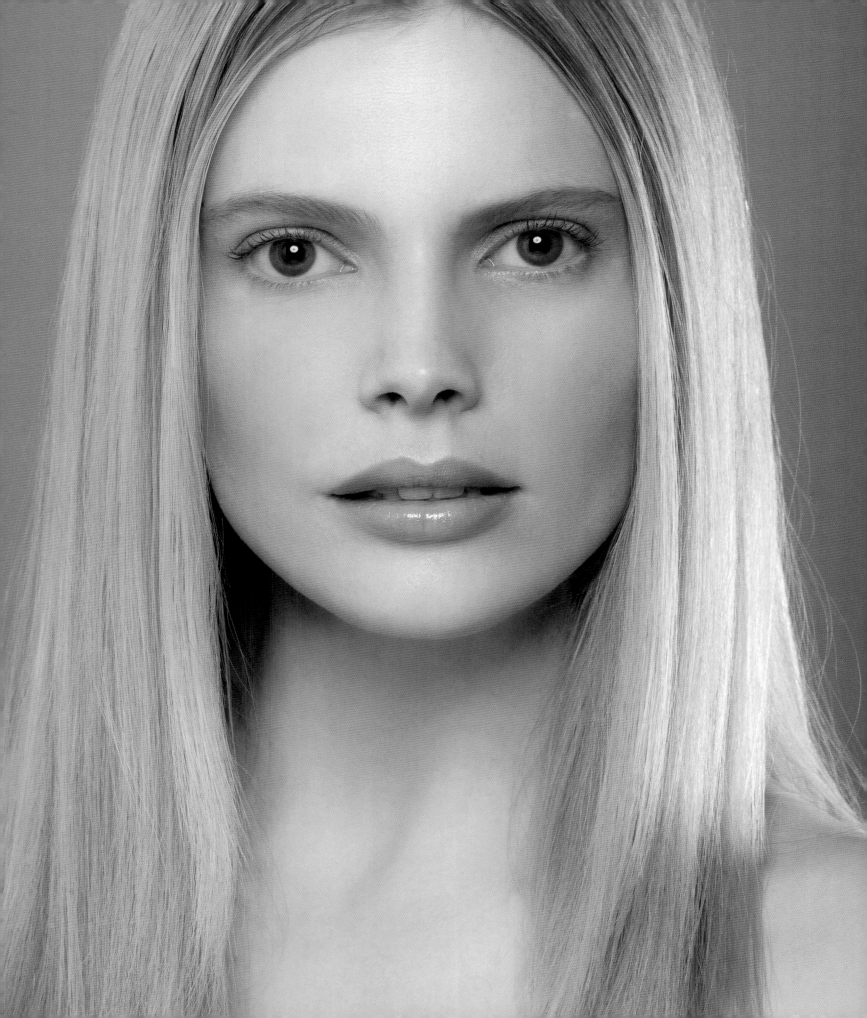

porcelain

The palest skin is incredibly sensitive to the sun, so wearing high SPF is crucial. Flawless porcelain skin is truly beautiful, but being the most translucent, it can also be the most difficult because blood vessels and capillaries show through the skin, making dark circles and imperfections noticeable. Unless you have freckles, your skin will have a cool pink undertone that is hard to warm up, so stick to pink-based foundation and cool colours. Use very pale blushes and avoid bronzers and fake tans, which will look too obvious. Celebrities with porcelain skin include Nicole Kidman, Kate Blanchett and Sophie Dahl.

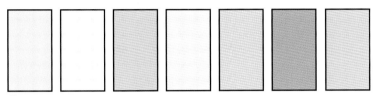

Eyes With porcelain skin, eyes are usually blue, green or hazel and are often prone to redness. Avoid heavy eyeliner and pink eyeshadows, which will emphasize this, and stick to cool neutrals or soft pastels. Shades of grey (ideal for eyeliner), blue and cool creams work well – go for darker shades within these families for the evening.

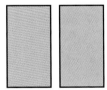

Cheeks Pale peach, apricot or very soft natural-blush pinks work well on porcelain skin, but don't go for anything too pink, as this will overemphasize the natural pink in your skin. Stick to a silvery highlighter on cheekbones.

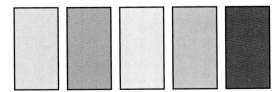

Lips Scarlet red looks beautiful with flawless porcelain skin, but it can be a hard look to pull off. Brownish pinks and soft apricots are more flattering for you than bubblegum pink.

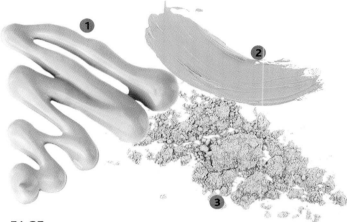

FACE

1 If your complexion is good, use a sheer tinted moisturizer, but if you need more coverage try a light fluid foundation – thick formulations will look like a mask. Choose a pale shade with 95 per cent pink tones. Make sure your foundation contains SPF 15, preferably higher.

2 A hydrating, creamy concealer is essential for the undereye area. Choose one with pink undertones to neutralize the blue circles.

3 Go for the sheerest translucent powder and only use it where you really need it.

TOP TIP

Be really careful of fake tan and bronzer. These products will invariably look too orange and fake on your skin. Try a tawny soft brown blush to bring warmth to your face instead.

fair

This is a very common skin tone for Caucasian women – the classic English rose complexion. Unlike porcelain skin, which tends to be more uniform, fair skin often has natural changes in tone across the face, with darker and lighter areas, rosy cheeks and sometimes freckles. Fair skin burns quite easily and is often prone to sensitivity, so SPF is an important component of daytime skincare and make-up. While the underlying skin tone is predominantly pink, there is some yellow, so you don't need to avoid pink colours entirely. Celebrities with fair skin include Cameron Diaz, Kate Winslett and Gwyneth Paltrow.

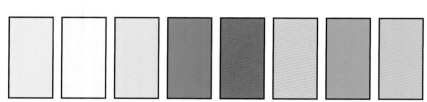

Eyes With a proportion of yellow in your skin tone as well as the dominant pink, you suit colours in both warm and cool tones. Eyes are darker, so you can wear deeper colours and stronger eyeliner than those with very pale eyes and skin. If you keep shades muted, it's hard to go wrong, although yellows and oranges won't suit you.

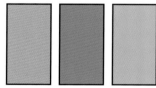

Cheeks Pink shades generally look lovely on fair skin – anything from brownish pink to fuchsia to fresh pink. Be careful with bronzer and avoid anything too dark or with too much orange or shimmer. Stay in silver tones for highlighter.

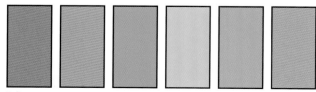

Lips Warm neutrals such as nudes and pinks are the most flattering. Finding the right shade of red can be difficult – you need one that's neither too blue-based nor too orange.

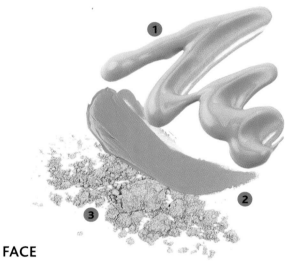

FACE

1 Colour-match your foundation carefully and be sure that it matches your neck. The right shade for you will be pink-based, but with a little warmth to it, especially in the summer when you may have a tan. Choose a foundation with at least SPF 15.

2 Dark undereye circles are often evident on fair skin and you may also be prone to redness around the nose and mouth. Choose a flesh-toned concealer with a creamy formulation to neutralize these problem areas.

3 If you need powder, keep it light and opt for an ultra-sheer finish.

TOP TIP

Sheer lipsticks or silky glosses will make darker lip colours more wearable for you.

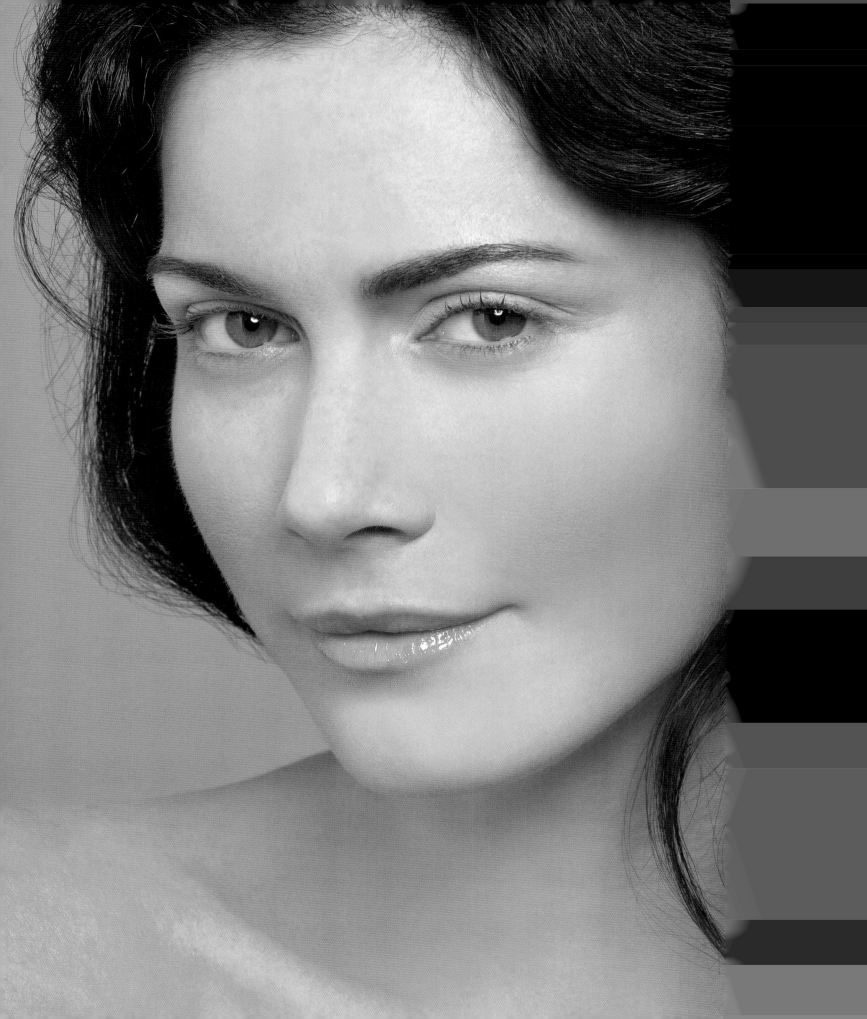

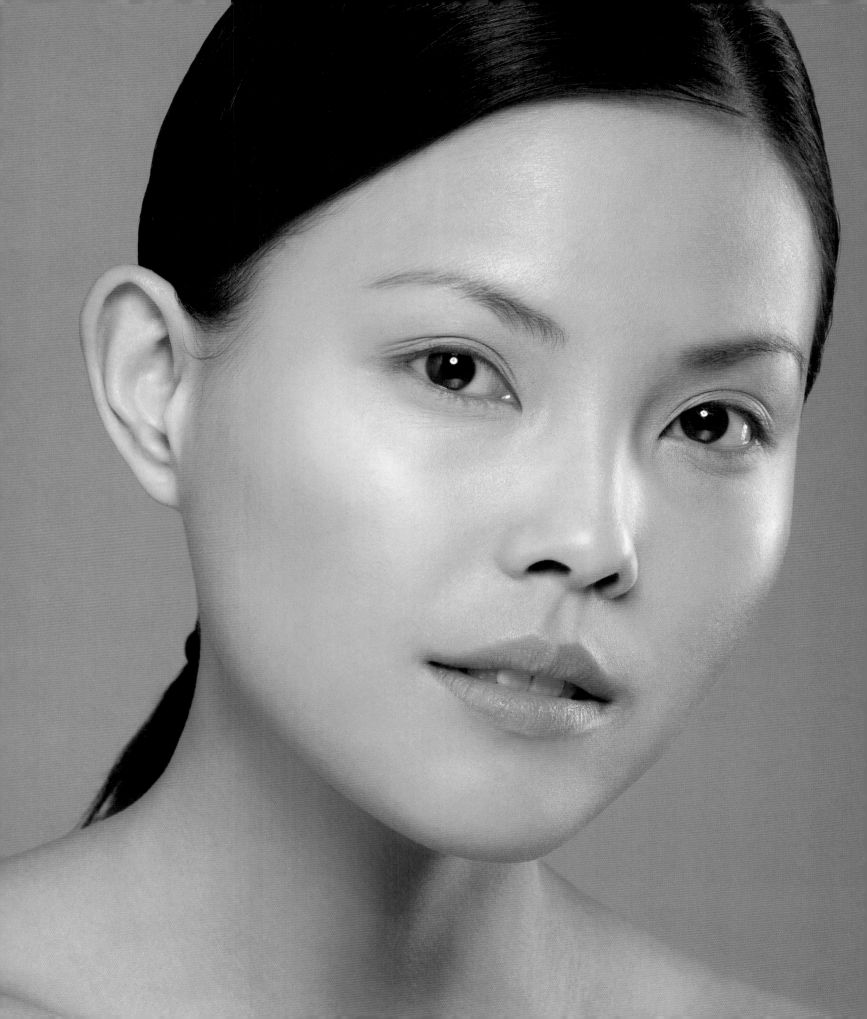

light olive

The direct counterpart to porcelain skin, light olive skin is predominantly yellow-toned but still very pale. The difference is that the yellow undertones make dark circles and blemishes less noticeable – skin looks somehow thicker and not so translucent. It is less likely to have the red pigmentation that is often a characteristic of pink-toned skin, so you can generally get away with lighter coverage. While pale olive skin tans more readily than porcelain skin, it still burns easily and should be protected with high SPF. Celebrities with light olive skin include Lucy Liu, Jennifer Aniston and Angelina Jolie.

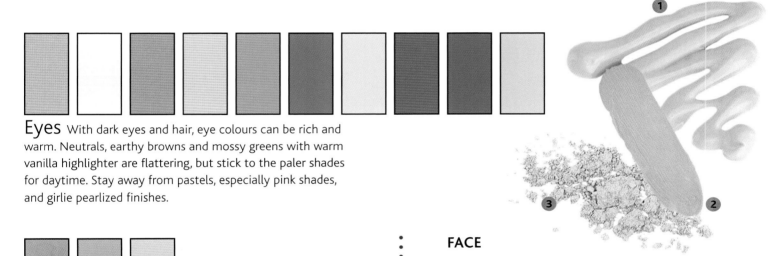

Eyes With dark eyes and hair, eye colours can be rich and warm. Neutrals, earthy browns and mossy greens with warm vanilla highlighter are flattering, but stick to the paler shades for daytime. Stay away from pastels, especially pink shades, and girlie pearlized finishes.

Cheeks Coral pinks and soft orange tones add warmth to the face. Because the skin is so pale, pinker tones that don't work on deep olive skin bring a pretty flush to the cheeks. Most bronzers, including pearlized ones, work well on light olive skin. To highlight the cheekbones, go for soft peach or gold tones.

Lips Most warm colours are flattering, such as coral and peachy pinks, and shades of berry, plum and brown. Go for orange undertones rather than blue, and stay away from fuchsia pink.

FACE

1 Foundation should be at least 95 per cent yellow with very little pink. Don't use one that is too dark for your natural colour.

2 Make sure that concealer is warm enough for your skin tone. Stay away from undereye brighteners that have pink tones and stick to a yellow base.

3 If your skin is very pale, you can get away with translucent powder, but if you go for anything darker, again make sure it has a yellow tone.

TOP TIP

While eye colours should be pale, going too pale on your lips can make you look washed out – choose a lip colour that's at least one shade darker than your skin.

dark olive

The typical skin type of Mediterranean countries, South America and parts of Asia, dark olive skin has a deep yellow tone. It tans very easily in the sun and stays tanned for longer than fair skin, but that doesn't mean that you should ignore sun protection – SPF should still be an important feature of your skincare regime, to protect your skin and delay the signs of ageing. In general, deep, rich, warm colours work well for you – shades lighter than your skin tone will drain you and make you look sallow. Celebrities with dark olive skin include Eva Longoria, Freida Pinto and Penélope Cruz.

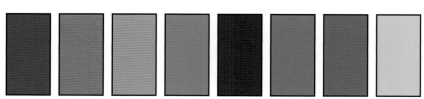

Eyes For a natural daytime look, go for warm gold, peach or olive green. For more drama, use deep purples, plums and greens, or rich golds and browns. Stay away from cool colours, especially silver and pale blue.

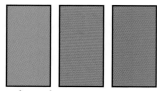

Cheeks Apricot and peachy pinks create a warm flush, while lighter plums and browns are also flattering. Bronzer works well for you – from warm gold to terracotta – including shimmery finishes. For highlighter, go for gold tones.

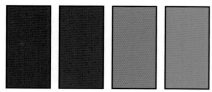

Lips Dark, warm colours work well on your lips, while pale colours will wash out your complexion. Shades of deep red, orange, coral, gold and brown look stunning, while deep fuchsia is striking and dramatic.

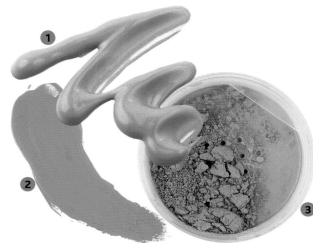

FACE

1 Your skin tone will probably be fairly even, so you won't need too much coverage. Tinted moisturizer works well on dark olive skin, for more coverage go for a yellow-based foundation.

2 Dark olive skin can be prone to oiliness and breakouts, so use a yellow-based concealer to cover blemishes.

3 If your skin tends to shine, use a fine yellow-toned powder.

TOP TIP

Smoky eyes in sultry neutrals – browns, bronzes, navy or charcoal – will play up your dark features. White and silver eyeshadows will make you look washed out.

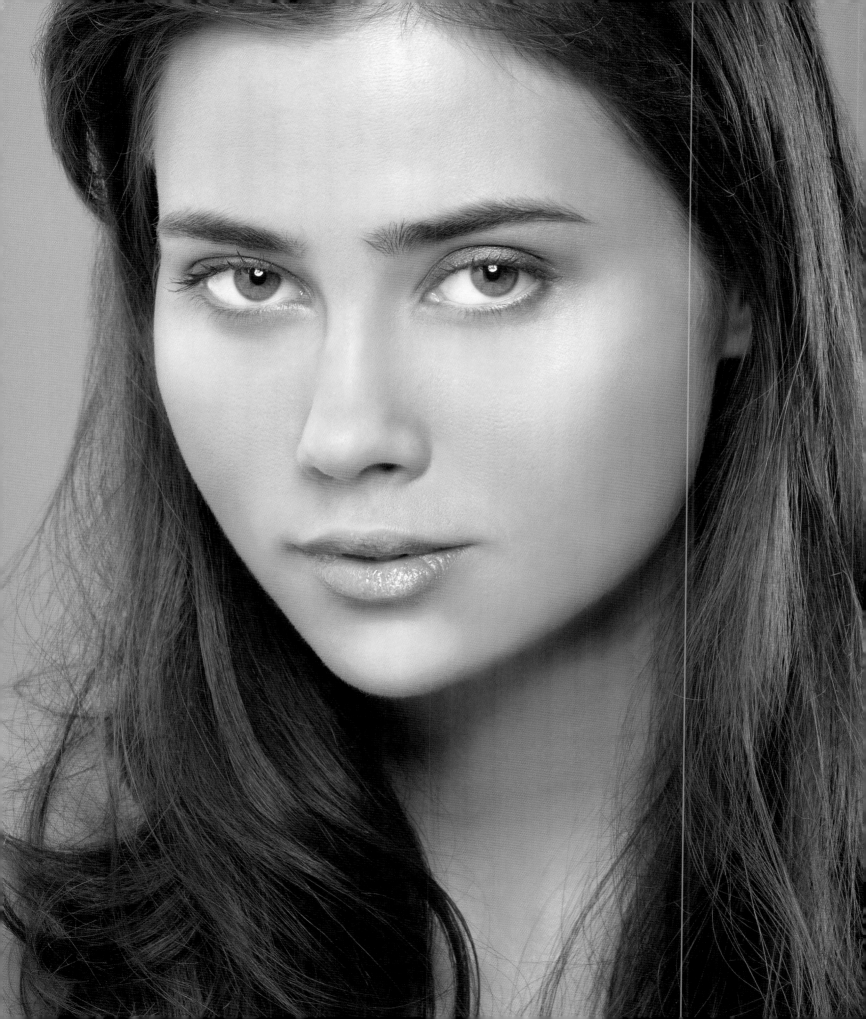

deep

Black skin can either have an olive or a red undertone. If your skin has olive tones, opt for rich warm shades to bring out the golden highlights. If you have red undertones, a cooler colour palette will be more flattering. In general, the deeper your skin, the darker and more dramatic the colours you can carry off on eyes, cheeks and lips, but remember to play up either the eyes or the lips, not both together. A wider range of colours tend to look good on you than on those with fairer skin, so have fun experimenting to see what suits you. Celebrities with deep skin include Halle Berry, Michelle Obama and Naomi Campbell.

Eyes If you have dark skin, try shades of bronze, burnt orange, emerald green, sapphire and plum. If your skin has a paler caramel tone, use olive green, warm gold, toffee and lighter plums. Shimmery and metallic textures are flattering for evening looks.

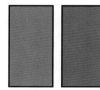

Cheeks If you have a cool skin tone, deep shades of plum and rose will look beautiful. Shades of apricot and bronzer are flattering on warm-toned skin, while deep gold highlighter will bring out the golden undertones.

Lips Most deep shades will work well on your lips, especially berry, rose, coral, bronze, terracotta, coffee and dark apricot. Glossy textures and gold add instant glamour.

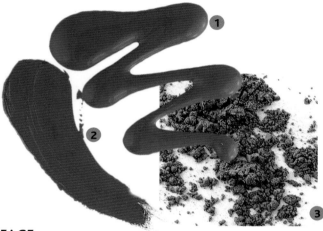

FACE

1 If you have red in your skin, choose a foundation with red undertones. If your skin contains olive, opt for a foundation with an ochre undertone.

2 To hide red thread veins or blemishes, use an olive-based concealer; to neutralize blue undereye circles choose a red-based concealer. For concealer that blends well with your skin, the same rule applies as for foundation.

3 To prevent your complexion from looking ashy, choose an ultra-fine powder in a dark shade that matches the undertone of your skin.

TOP TIP

Black skin is less likely to burn than fairer skin, but you should still wear SPF in warmer weather to prevent fine lines and pigmentation.

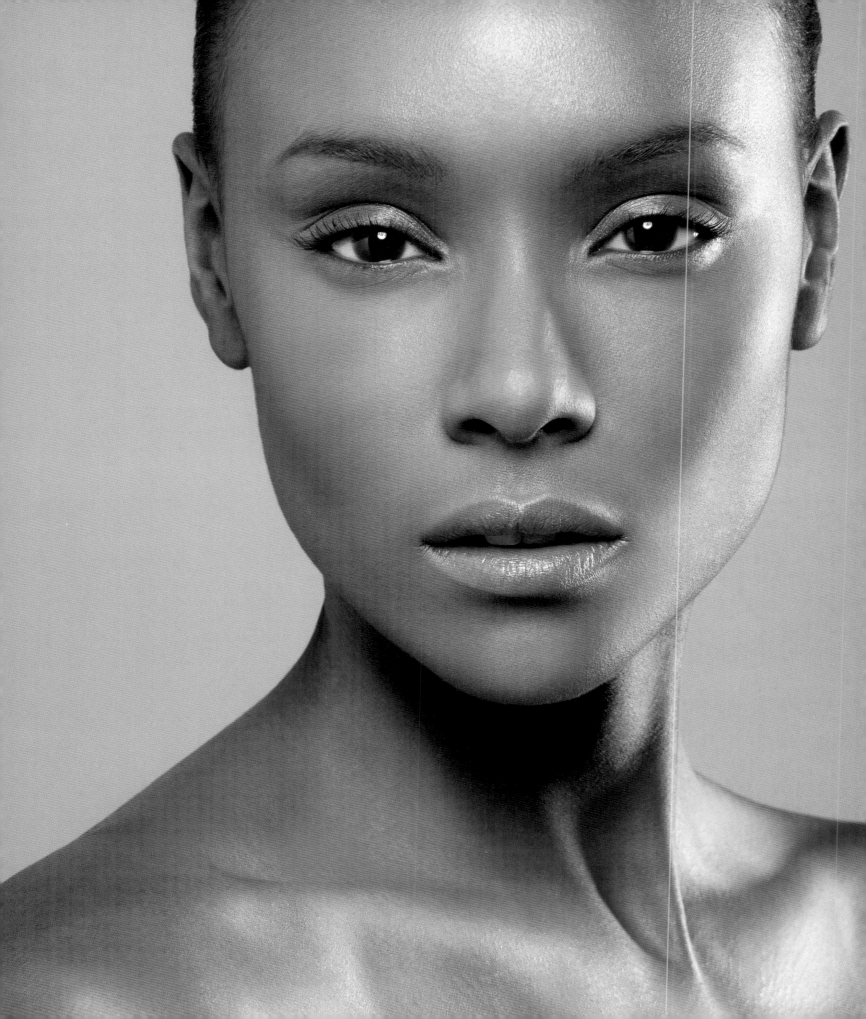

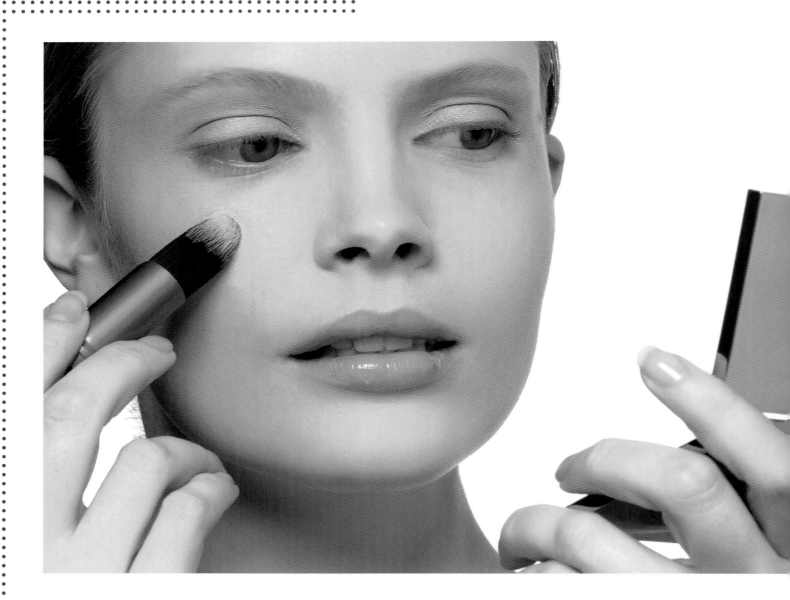

BEAUTIFUL AT ANY AGE

Make-up can't turn back time, but it can enhance natural beauty at any age. Update the textures and colours of the make-up you use and how you apply it to make the best of your features and disguise signs of ageing.

Although many mature women wouldn't dream of squeezing into the miniskirts or boob tubes they wore in their youth, they are more than happy to continue wearing the same make-up. Begin your update by investigating the new colours and textures available and trying them out to see what looks most flattering. Remember: don't let your make-up define you – use it to show your features to their best advantage.

My secret Always apply make-up in as much natural light as possible and use a good mirror.

Looking young for longer

» 90 per cent of the ageing process can be traced back to sun exposure, so always wear a minimum of SPF 15.

» Mature skin dehydrates easily, making lines more prominent. Use a gentle cleanser, rich moisturizer and a hydrating serum.

» Drink plenty of water and refresh the skin with a mineral spray.

» Fish oils, fruit and vegetables keep the skin looking youthful, while cigarettes, alcohol and caffeine have a negative effect.

» As you age, reap the benefits of 'smart' make-up, which is full of active antiageing ingredients.

Regain the plump skin of youth

As we age, the skin's collagen and elastin production slows down. These are what help to give skin its plumpness and elasticity, and without them it becomes more prone to wrinkles and sagging. Here are some tips to keep skin looking its best.

Face

» Use a moisture-boosting mask twice a week and apply moisturizer morning and evening.
» Serums are a great 'pick me up' and deliver a lot of moisture. Pat the serum into the skin and let it sink in for five minutes, then apply moisturizer.
» Choose a foundation that contains ingredients to plump and smooth.

Eyes

» The sensitive skin around the eyes is most prone to lines, so use an eye cream or gel with an SPF during the day.
» Eye creams or serums applied at night nourish the skin while you are sleeping.

Lips

» A moisturizing lip cream that boosts collagen production will keep lips hydrated.
» Avoid plumping lipglosses that literally sting the lips, as these can be very drying.
» Drink water – dehydration leads to dry skin and chapped lips.

Take off ten years with make-up

There are a few typical beauty complaints that come with age – skin looks duller, fine lines and wrinkles appear around eyes and lips, and brows and lashes may get sparser. These simple make-up tricks can take off ten years.

Skin

» Skin thins as you get older, so use lighter coverage – heavy foundation collects in wrinkles, drawing attention to them. Tinted moisturizers, mousses, light liquid or crème compact foundations give sheer coverage and absorb well.
» Use foundation sparingly, just where you really need it. Choose light-reflecting formulations.
» If you need powder for oil control, choose translucent talc-free powder with light-reflecting particles, or use blotting tissues. Mattifying products can make mature skin look dry.

Eyes

» To cover dark undereye circles use a pink-toned concealer. Dab a creamy textured yellow-toned concealer on top, matching the colour to the rest of the face.
» A neutral palette of brown, taupe, beige, peach and soft pinks is more flattering for mature skin. Blending is key, so invest in good brushes.
» Opt for soft brown or grey mascaras and eyeliners, as black can be harsh. Apply mascara to the upper lashes only and don't overload them.
» Once you are over 50, steer clear of liquid eyeliner, which can feather into the fine lines.

My secret Choose colours that look natural against your skin in rich, hydrating formulas: crème blush, crème

» To make eyelashes appear thicker, work dark brown pencil eyeliner between the roots, then go over it with a dark shadow and smudge gently.

» Use an eyebrow pencil in the exact shade of your brows to fill in any gaps with light feathery strokes, then apply a little brow powder.

Cheeks

» A touch of blush on the apple of the cheeks draws attention away from drooping eyes and adds warmth.

» Apply blush only to the apples of the cheeks. With age, the face becomes thinner and applying blush to the bones exaggerates this.

» Use moisturizing crème products rather than powder blush, and blend thoroughly.

» Warm bronze or peach blushes are more flattering than bright pinks.

Lips

» Lipstick will often bleed into the fine lines around the mouth, so apply a waxy lipliner to seal the lip. Draw the outline first, then smile to stretch your lips and reapply. Don't draw outside your natural lip line. Apply a little translucent powder around the lip to set the colour.

» Sheer finishes look more flattering than matte. Always choose a moisturizing or hydrating formulation.

» Dark colours minimize lips, whereas a lighter, shimmering colour makes lips look fuller. A dab of gloss at the centre of the lower lip gives a fuller pout.

» For a glossy finish, either mix balm with your favourite lip colour or try a lip stain layered with a dab of gloss.

Smoothing out fine lines

» Use primer under foundation to provide a smoother surface for make-up.

» Avoid thick foundation and powder as they sink into lines and make them more obvious.

» A highlighter can disguise deeper lines – use soft pearl colours, but avoid frosty shades, which will draw attention to the lines.

» Use a mattifying gel on lines above the lip. The silicone will fill out the lines and make them less noticeable.

» Use a waxy lipliner to prevent lipstick from bleeding. Antifeathering lipsticks are also available.

eyeshadow and moisture-rich foundation. Vibrant or contrasting colours can be very ageing.

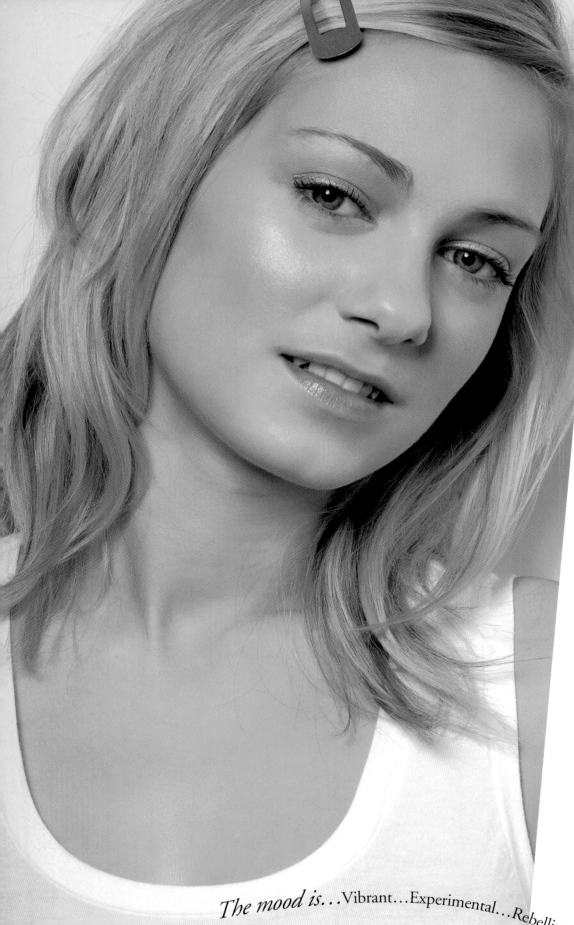

teens to early 20s

Almost nothing is off limits make-up wise, so enjoy bright, provocative colours and expressive textures, and be confident in the way you look. This is the period in your life to find and create your identity, so make-up can be vibrant, moody, experimental or rebellious.

For the eyes, a single line of glittery gel liner in a contrasting colour looks fresh and pretty. Here, turquoise gel liner along the top lid gives a burst of colour to an otherwise soft, natural look, with gently flushed cheeks and pale pink lightly glossy lips.

TOP TIP

Apply moisturizer and eye cream at night, and use a lighter moisturizer with sunscreen during the day. Getting into good habits as a teenager and carrying them through your 20s will do more to keep your skin looking younger longer than any number of expensive creams applied later.

*The mood is…*Vibrant…Experimental…Rebellious…Provocative…Expressive…Jubilant

mid 20s to 30s

This is often a time when you strive for sophistication and try to appear more grown-up in order to be taken seriously. Make-up is often trend-led – image is all.

Fresh and firm skin means that there are no limitations – all the textures that are tricky for older skin still work perfectly. Frost or glitter finishes look great – in moderation, of course. Styles like a 1950s flick or bold blocks of colour are hard to do successfully if the eyelid droops or if you have wrinkles, so the joy of being young means you can have lots of fun with eyeliner.

Now is the time to discover neutrals, but to accessorize them with colour. For day, instead of wearing plain neutrals on the eye, choose a shimmery texture, with sheer colour on the cheeks and glossy lips.

TOP TIP
Shiny metallics on your lids can be lots of fun. Make up your own metallic eyeshadow with a high-shimmer pigment and Vaseline.

*The mood is…*Fashionable…Aspirational…Sophisticated…Grown-up…Fun…Fresh

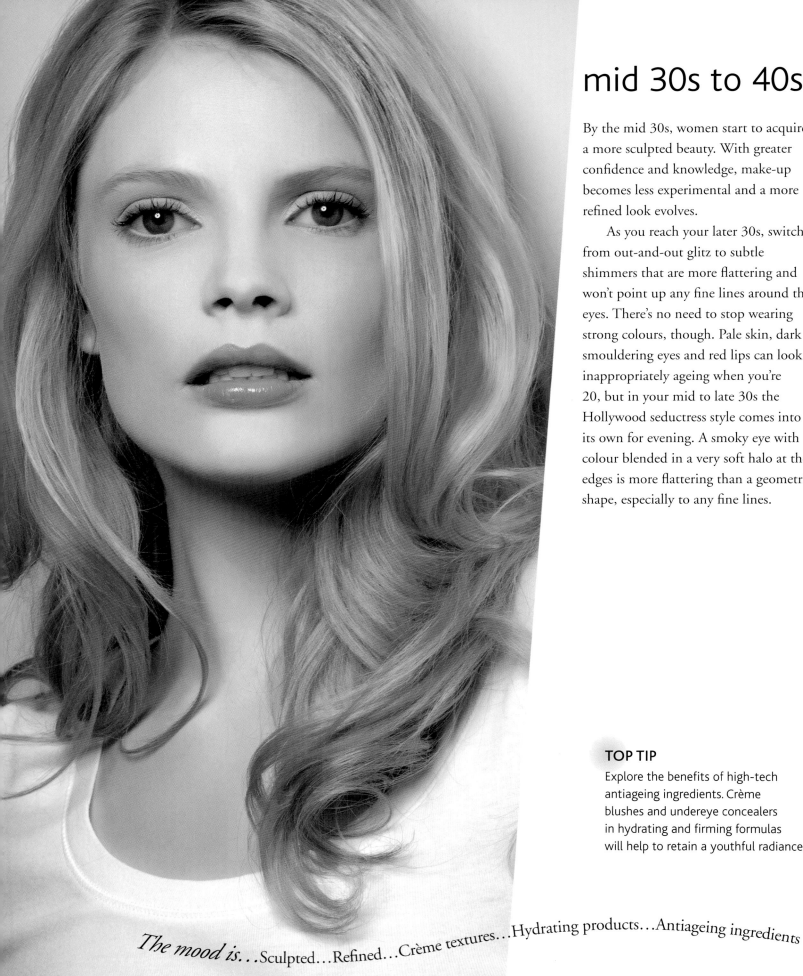

mid 30s to 40s

By the mid 30s, women start to acquire a more sculpted beauty. With greater confidence and knowledge, make-up becomes less experimental and a more refined look evolves.

As you reach your later 30s, switch from out-and-out glitz to subtle shimmers that are more flattering and won't point up any fine lines around the eyes. There's no need to stop wearing strong colours, though. Pale skin, dark smouldering eyes and red lips can look inappropriately ageing when you're 20, but in your mid to late 30s the Hollywood seductress style comes into its own for evening. A smoky eye with colour blended in a very soft halo at the edges is more flattering than a geometric shape, especially to any fine lines.

TOP TIP

Explore the benefits of high-tech antiageing ingredients. Crème blushes and undereye concealers in hydrating and firming formulas will help to retain a youthful radiance.

The mood is…Sculpted…Refined…Crème textures…Hydrating products…Antiageing ingredients

the 40s

Signs of ageing start to show as less collagen is produced and skin loses its elasticity, so firming and antiageing ingredients become vital allies. The emphasis is on bringing back the skin's youthful glow, so look for a creamy light-reflecting foundation. Brows may become sparser, so define them to add structure to the face, and use a lip pencil to redefine the lip shape.

Switch black mascara for brown, for a softer look. Restrict colour to a palette you know suits you. There are beautiful shades of plum, brown, green and grey that are flattering no matter what your age, but pinks, yellows and blues can be difficult to wear. Stay away from frosted metallics.

TOP TIPS

» Moisturize well and use an eye cream. Try a face oil after cleansing.

» Wear a radiance crème for day and layer it with foundation for night.

» Powder can dry the skin, but an ultra-fine powder with light-reflecting particles controls shine while adding luminosity.

» Dark undereye circles are less easy to cover. Use a creamy concealer to counteract the underlying blue.

» Crème blush is great for dry skin. Beige and apricot are elegant and fresh.

» Use a waxy lipliner to stop lipstick from bleeding. Or, just use a lip stain with a touch of gloss.

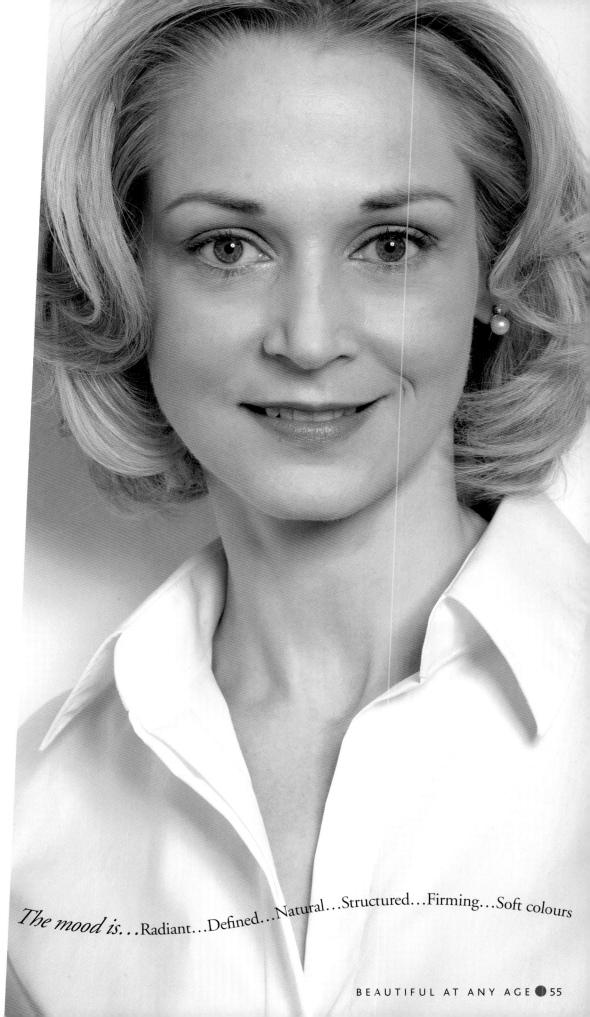

The mood is...Radiant...Defined...Natural...Structured...Firming...Soft colours

the 50s

While it is wise to stick to a neutral palette, new technology means that powder, sparkling and metallic formulations are finer than ever before and can be worn by older women without being ageing. Beware of pearl and high-shimmer make-up as these intensify the appearance of fine lines. Matte textures can make the skin look dull, so choose light-reflecting powder and iridescent finishes to create a soft effect.

Care for your skin with very gentle cleansers and rich moisturizers. You may find that with the menopause your skin changes – it may become very dry or have oily patches that can lead to blemishes. Treat dry areas with a rich cream or facial oil. Oily areas can be very frustrating, but don't resort to harsh cleansers and use an oil-free water-based cream.

TOP TIPS

» Choose light-reflecting, skin-brightening formulations.

» Keep your skin hydrated and exfoliated, and treat yourself to facials.

» For your eyes, use a palette of soft, warm colours. Apply a neutral base over the lid and socket. Intensify colour at the socket to open up your eyes – the skin on the upper lid can sag slightly, so blend the socket colour up so that you can see it when the eye is open.

» Bright red lipsticks are usually too harsh. I prefer a lip stain with a touch of gloss.

*The mood is...*Neutral palette...Renewed sparkle...Fine metallics...Iridescent finishes...Halo effect

the 60s and beyond

By the 60s, a woman has learnt to embrace and respect the maturity that comes with age – lines and furrows can be celebrated as the map of a life well lived.

Mature skin loses colour and you must change foundation shade to take account of this. Choose light-reflecting formulations and, for extra radiance, add illuminator to foundation. Liquids and mousses give very sheer coverage and won't look powdery or crease. For even coverage, gently work the foundation into wrinkles by slightly stretching the skin. Use a crème blush in a gentle peach or warm bronze to add healthy colour to the apples of the cheeks, and top with a light dusting of fine skin-brightening powder. Browns, peaches and soft pinks are flattering to mature skin. Heavy colours tend to crease in the eye, so try gentler shades and spend time layering colour with a good brush to make it last longer and adhere better.

TOP TIPS

» Cleanse the face using a muslin cloth and alternating hot and cold water. This gently exfoliates while stimulating blood flow for a brighter complexion.

» Use facial oil under moisturizer for a boost of hydration.

» To cover dark circles or age spots, apply concealer with a brush and blend with your finger or a sponge.

» Highlight the eye in a neutral colour, then add a soft brown at the lash line and blend up. Line the inner rim of the lower lid with white for brighter eyes.

» Strong lipstick can be ageing, so for a softer, sheer look, mix your favourite lipstick with balm, or use a natural pencil with gloss.

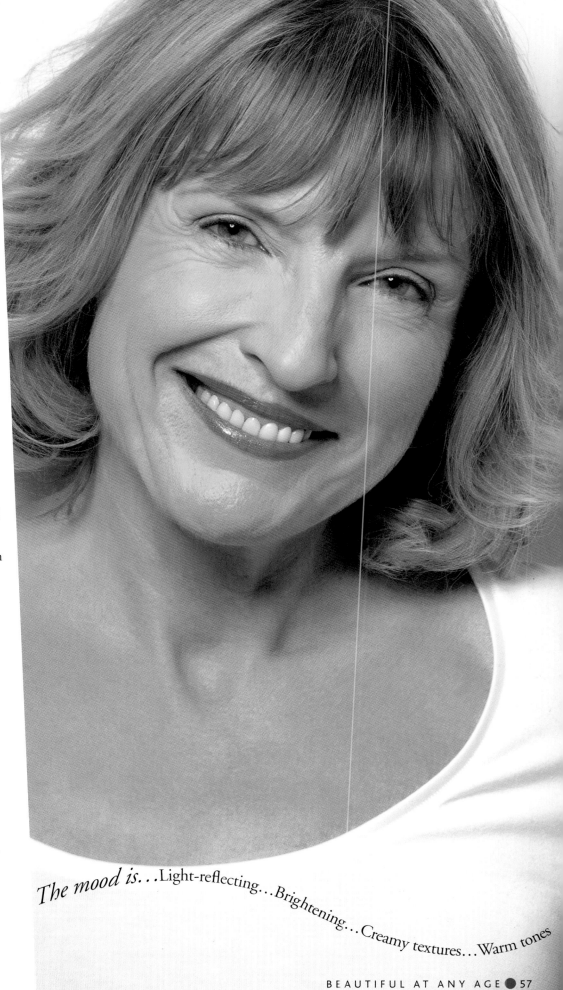

The mood is…Light-reflecting…Brightening…Creamy textures…Warm tones

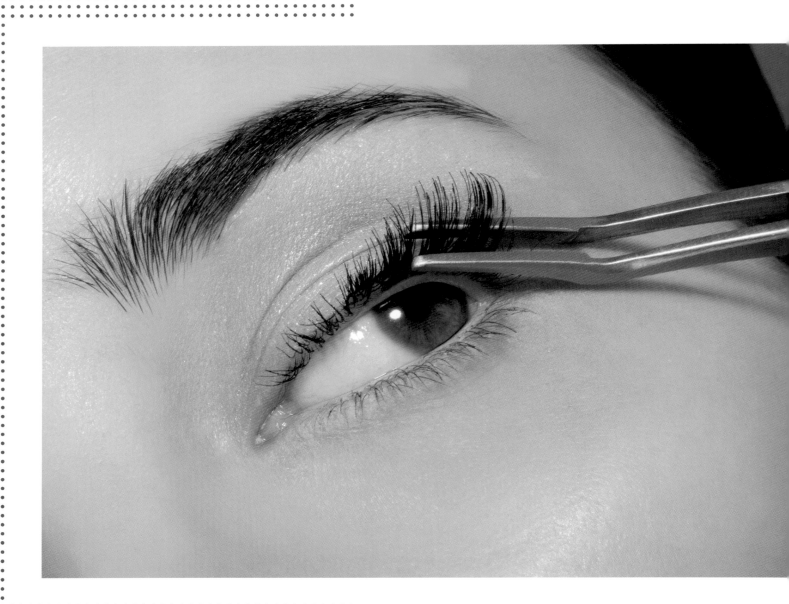

TOOLS OF THE TRADE

Using the right tools is key to achieving professional results. Make-up is expensive, and while it may seem extravagant to invest in all the kit, it will ensure you always get the most out of your products.

Applying make-up correctly with the appropriate tool gives a longer-lasting finish, greater precision and more natural results. Foundation, concealer and powder will appear to sink into the skin seamlessly, lips and eyes will be defined more accurately and colours will blend perfectly.

As a professional make-up artist, I have an enormous collection of brushes of all shapes, sizes and textures, not to mention tweezers, lash curlers and separators – the list is endless. What you choose to include in your make-up kit will depend to a great extent on the make-up textures you prefer. As a rule, synthetic brushes should be used to blend crème and liquid formulations, while natural brushes are best for powders. The other thing to consider is how 'hands on' you like to be. Many women prefer to apply foundation, concealer and crème blush with their fingertips, as they find that the warmth of their fingers makes the product more workable.

TOP TIPS

» Always choose a good-quality brush to avoid moulting.

» A brush with a short handle lets you get closer to the face and maintain better control.

KEEP IT CLEAN Good hygiene is crucial to avoid breakouts and eye infections.

» Cleanse your skin before applying make-up and remove it thoroughly at the end of the day (see pages 28–31).

» If you apply make-up with your fingers, wash your hands first.

» Don't share eyeliners, mascaras or lipsticks, to avoid spreading infections.

» Wash your brushes using brush cleanser or mild shampoo, working thoroughly between the fibres. Rinse and squeeze gently in a towel. Leave to dry over the side of the sink, so that air can circulate around the fibres. Only ever air-dry your brushes; a hairdryer will damage them.

Synthetic brushes, which are easier to clean, should be used to blend crème and liquid formulations, while natural brushes, which are softer on the skin, are best for powders.'

essential tool kit

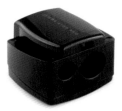

Here's a selection of what I consider to be the most essential make-up tools. If you invest in them all, you will have covered all bases, but feel free to pick and choose depending on personal preference.

Pencil sharpener
Buy a good-quality one with two openings to sharpen fat eye crayons as well as thinner lip and eye pencils.

Fine cotton buds
Dip the tip in make-up remover or foundation to clean up smudges or mistakes.

Lash curlers
Curling your lashes makes them look longer and opens up the eye. Use this invaluable tool before applying mascara.

False-lash applicator and glue
False lashes create instant glamour, but it's easy to apply them badly so that they look obvious. Use the applicator as a clip to hold the lash firmly as you apply glue along the strip, then attach the lash, pressing the curve all the way along the lid to stick evenly.

Lash separator
Use after applying mascara to eliminate clogging. Simply work the tool between the lashes to separate them.

Eyebrow brush/comb
Neat, defined eyebrows frame the face and can be your personal signature.

Tweezers
Essential for good grooming, tweezers can be used to keep unruly brows neat.

'It may seem extravagant to kit yourself out with an array of brushes and other gadgets, but it will be a good investment in the long run, as they will ensure you are always able to get the most out of your products.'

1 Lipstick/brow/crème eyeshadow brush
Use this square-topped brush to line and fill in your lips and eyes and to define your brows. The most multipurpose brush of all, the densely packed nylon bristles are easy to clean and stiff enough to create a precise line. The best quality feel firm, but never scratchy or hard.

2 Powder eyeshadow brush
Use a medium-sized brush to apply powder eyeshadow to the entire lid and for detailing certain areas. The densely packed 100 per cent natural hair is soft and easy to blend with. The brush should be no bigger than the eyelid itself.

3 Smudging brush
Use to diffuse eyeshadow across the eyelid. The deep brush is cut to fit the eye socket, making precise application and blending simple.

4 Concealer/crème eyeshadow brush
This synthetic-bristle brush has a pointed tip to conceal with precision. Use it to apply and smooth concealer around the eye area and over blemishes, and to apply crème eyeshadow.

5 Pointed eyeshadow brush
Use a detail and depth brush under the eye and to blend eyeshadow in corners and creases.

6 Pointed foundation brush
If you use any foundation that requires a good deal of working into the skin – mineral powder or crème – a foundation brush is essential. It allows you to blend the product without risking getting dirt onto your face. It gives good control and makes it easy to get to hard-to-reach places around the eye cavity. The pointed synthetic head applies just the right amount of pressure to help minimize imperfections and is easier to clean than natural fibres.

7 Blush brush
The gently curved top follows the contours and bone structure of cheeks and temples, allowing you to blend colour evenly without streaking. Use it to sculpt areas of the face with precision.

8 Powder or bronzer brush
A large dense brush made with 100 per cent natural hair allows perfect application and blending. Use this brush to smooth and polish powder over the face for a natural finish.

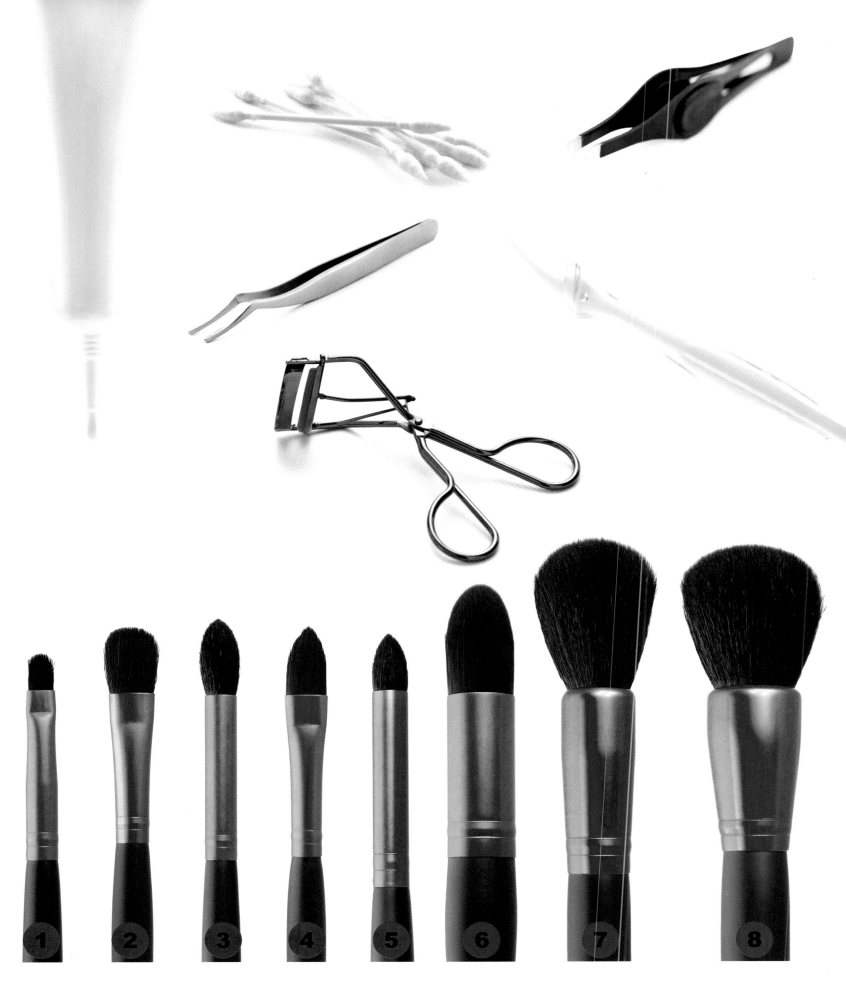

WONDER PRODUCTS & BEAUTY BUZZWORDS

With new products launching every season, choosing the best ones for you can be daunting. It's easy to be seduced by the hype and to end up with a bathroom shelf and make-up bag brimming with expensive creams and cosmetics that are not right for you.

The groundbreaking advances that have been made in the beauty industry over the past decade are undeniable. Formulations are more refined and ingredients more high-tech and specific than ever before, so whatever your priorities and concerns, you will find an array of products to target every one. The secret in negotiating your way through this raft of wonder products is to know your skin and to learn how it responds, both to the environment and to what you put on it, and to make informed choices based on its specific requirements and on your lifestyle. Natural ingredients may be essential for your peace of mind, for example, while two-in-one 'smart' products could allow you to cut corners when you have a busy schedule.

Of course, it is not just what you put on your skin that counts, but also what you feed it with. A healthy, balanced diet rich in fruit and vegetables is essential to provide the nutrients the skin needs to repair and regenerate, while drinking plenty of water helps to flush out toxins and keeps the skin hydrated.

Miracle-working ingredients and buzzwords to look for:

» *Vitamins,* particularly A, C and E, which boost the skin's defences and keep it healthy and strong.

» *Antioxidants,* which help to fight the damaging effects of free radicals and other environmental pollutants.

» *Omega-rich oils,* which keep the skin supple, nourished and in peak condition.

» *Peptides,* which encourage the skin to produce more collagen.

» *Retinyl palmitate,* which aids cell renewal and smooths skin.

» *SPF 15* – for any product worn on the face during the day, SPF 15 or higher is essential.

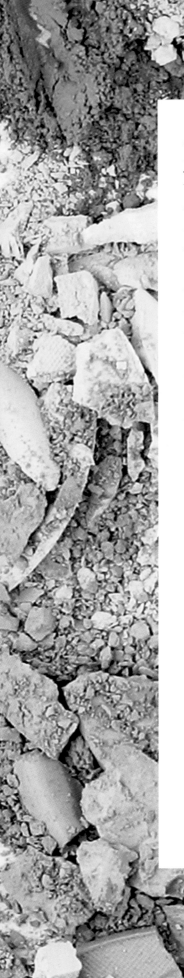

Organic products

Just as we worry about what we eat, it's natural to worry about what we put on our skin. There are some excellent 100 per cent toxin-free skincare and make-up ranges that give great results without compromising on ingredients.

Dr Hauschka has good foundations and a bronze concentrate that can be mixed with moisturizer to subtly even skin tone, soften blemishes and give a sunkissed finish.

Green People created Britain's first organic lipstick, which contains fabulous moisturizing ingredients, while There Must Be a Better Way produces lovely lip crèmes.

Other companies that offer a good range of organic make-up are Australian brand Nvey Eco and The Organic Pharmacy, while Living Nature makes a great mascara formulated not to irritate sensitive eyes. Other favourite organic brands are Ren, Aesop and Aveda.

'Smart' products

So-called 'smart' make-up that combines the technology and ingredients of antiageing skincare with luxury make-up formulations is the new kid on the beauty industry block. Lipsticks and glosses that plump your pout to bee-stung proportions, as well as hydrate and protect; foundations that combine not only SPF and antioxidants, but also ingredients that stimulate the production of collagen, encourage cell renewal and help to smooth out fine lines; undereye concealers that hydrate the delicate eye area while covering dark shadows; and medicated concealers that heal blemishes as well as hide them. These products represent a leap forward in terms of two-in-one products and provide an extra boost to your skin throughout the day.

Mineral make-up

This has been the biggest new story in cosmetics for years. It is light, long-lasting and great for sensitive or acne-prone skin, but it requires a slightly different application technique.

PREPARE Unless your skin is extremely oily, moisturize before applying foundation. Mineral make-up relies on the skin's oils to absorb it, and without them it sits on the surface.

TOOLS Mineral make-up needs to be worked into the skin, so make sure your brush is good quality with dense firm bristles that are comfortable on the skin. The short handle and shaped bristles of a kabuki brush let you get close to the face and into awkward corners around the nose and eyes.

APPLY Don't overload the brush, tap away any excess and then work the brush on the skin in small circular motions, paying special attention to creases around the nose. Think of polishing a table – the trick is not to add more polish, but to work the initial quantity until it covers the whole area.

BLUSH Apply as you would a normal powder blush, but work it into the skin well to be sure it is properly absorbed and blended. A trick is to spritz your brush very lightly with water before working the blush – it can help blush to last longer, but you need to be careful as it's easy to make the blush too liquid and spread it too far.

EYES The benefit of most mineral eyeshadows is that they can be applied wet or dry. Use a normal dense brush to apply colour on the lid, or wet an angled brush and use the eyeshadow as an eyeliner. When using the eyeshadow dry, work the colour into the lid with mini-polishing movements. Once again, start with a little and apply more only as you need it.

THE NEW NO-RULE BEAUTY RULES The new products that fill our make-up bags allow us to be a lot freer. Here are my five top tips:

Eyes Layering different textures is a boon of new formulations. I use crème eyeshadow and then dust with a powder eyeshadow in a toning shade for depth of colour.

Skin Apply foundation only where you need it. Modern foundations sink into the skin so well that you just need touches, mainly on the cheeks and nose, to even out colour.

Cheeks Apply blush high, blending out towards the ear to elongate the cheekbone, or on the apple of the cheeks, for a flush of colour.

Lips Stain is a great invention. Apply stain to bare lips and then use a pencil to sculpt on top. The undertone of colour peeps through, giving a depth of hue on an otherwise nude lip.

Don't follow rules! Learn the shape and structure of your face, then just have fun doing what looks right.

MAKE-UP MOT

As the seasons change, refresh your make-up bag to keep up with new trends and to make sure your make-up stays clean and hygienic.

Make-up and skincare products past their use-by date can harbour bacteria that put your health and beauty at risk. In addition, the type of products you wear as well as the colours you choose will alter from summer to winter. Many women need no persuading to try out new colours and textures, but they are less willing to throw away a favourite lipstick that's been nestling at the bottom of their make-up bag for years, or an eyeshadow bought for a party on Millennium Eve. Cosmetics are expensive, and while we readily throw away food that's past its use-by date, many of us hang onto make-up for years, often sharing it and applying it in ways that can make us vulnerable to infections. Throwing away half-used products may hurt, but detoxing your make-up bag is the perfect excuse to discover some new favourites.

It should make us pause for thought when we realize that foundation and skincare products are absorbed by the skin, while lipstick is ingested when we eat and drink. A mascara wand can foster bacteria that cause conjunctivitis and the pumping action pushes them deep into the product – if mascara is shared, the spread of infection is inevitable. If you do get an eye infection or a coldsore, throw away any product that's been used on the offending area, and wash the brush every time you apply concealer to a spot. Avoid using the sponges that come with foundation or powder compacts, as these transfer bacteria directly between the face and the product.

GUIDE TO MAKE-UP EXPIRATION

EU legislation requires cosmetics to be labelled with a date of minimum durability, but there is no definition of how long a product remains usable. Keep the lids on tightly and store away from heat.

3–6 MONTHS mascara
6–8 MONTHS concealer, cleanser, crème foundation, liquid foundation, moisturizer
1 YEAR blush, eyeshadow, lipgloss, lipstick, loose powder, pressed powder, shimmer powder, toner
18 MONTHS eye and lip pencils

CLEAR OUT THE CLUTTER

Empty your make-up bag. If it's in good condition, put it through the washing machine; if it has seen better days, throw it out and buy a new one.

Wash brushes with mild shampoo and clean tweezers, lash curlers and pencil sharpeners by wiping with a few drops of tea-tree essential oil.

Replace mascara every three months or so. Regularly clean the wand to prevent it from becoming clogged with product.

Throw away dried-up products or any that smell or taste bad. Wax-based cosmetics are less likely to harbour bacteria than liquid or oil-based products. Be ruthless about any products you never wear.

Sharpen all eye and lip pencils and make sure they have a lid that fits. Sharpening not only ensures precise application, but also removes the top layer, which might be dirty.

Reward yourself with a new lip or eye colour so that you don't get stuck in a style rut. At the start of each season, highlight the new colours and products that look set to make a stir.

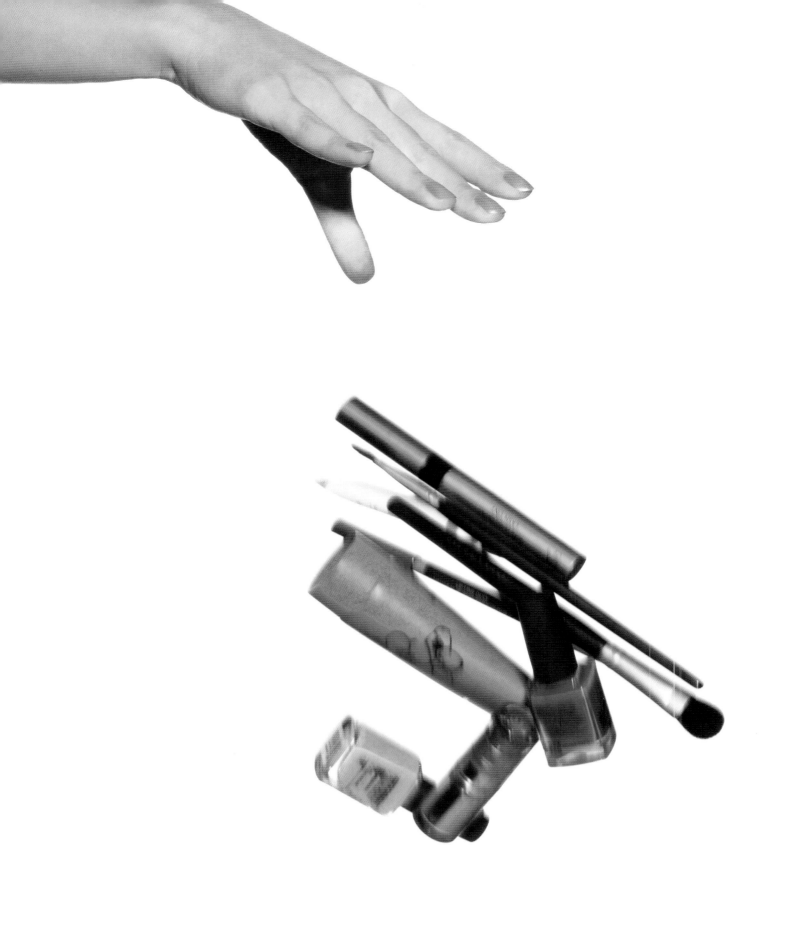

spring/summer

When the weather heats up, it can be hard to stay looking your best. You need to protect your skin from the sun and prevent it from drying out in the air-con, but any heavy product you use to help with those problems can leave skin looking greasy. In addition, you want make-up that looks natural but stays on all day, so you look cool and lovely all summer.

Protection and hydration

Sit in the shade where possible and wear a hat and sunglasses. Keep skin hydrated and protected with a booster serum and an oil-free moisturizer with SPF. You may prefer to use an additional block to protect your skin from UV and pollution, such as Clinique City-Block, which acts as a primer to help foundation to stay on longer and feels very light on the skin.

Light long-lasting make-up

FACE Summer calls for a sheer finish, so switch to a tinted moisturizer or a liquid foundation and use it only on the areas where you need it. Heavy foundations not only slide and crease in warm weather, but also feel uncomfortable and require powder to set them. Powder mineral foundation is fantastic for oily skin, as it helps to absorb oils and contains SPF. If you tan easily, you may need a darker shade in the summer to avoid a 'pale mask' effect.

Any compact foundation being 'retired' until winter should be wiped with a clean sponge and covered with plastic or paper. Make sure the lid is tightly closed.

QUICK FIX Properly applied foundation should last most of the day. Mop up shine with blotting tissues and, if necessary, dab a touch more liquid foundation onto key areas. If you have used powder, you won't be able to do this, so keep your look as light as possible.

EYES Groomed brows give the most natural look a certain polish. Pluck any stray hairs two or three times a week and trim any that are too long. Then spritz hairspray onto your eyebrow comb and set.

Keep a neutral eyeshadow palette in your make-up bag and treat yourself to one or two new colours, then master a new style (see overleaf for inspiration). Use light, natural eyeshadow with a touch of shimmer for daytime and apply mascara only on the upper lashes to avoid panda eyes. Lash tint or waterproof mascara last better in the heat. Give black eyeliner a rest until autumn and use a neutral brown instead, or try blue or jade for a colourful change.

QUICK FIX Carry a cotton bud with you to clean up any smudging under the eyes. Well-applied shadow won't crease, but it may wear off.

CHEEKS Powder blush can feel too heavy in summer, so put it away until winter. Crème colour can slide in heat, but it looks natural outdoors and in summer light. Or, use a stain or a creamy bronzing powder, which sinks into skin rather than sitting on top.

QUICK FIX Keep a bronzing compact in your bag so that you can touch up your eyes or sculpt your cheekbones to create a glamorous look while you're out and about.

LIPS Sheer balms and glosses look more summery and natural than heavy lipsticks that stay on all day, but they need to be reapplied frequently. Kill two birds with one stone by using a sheer balm that contains SPF to care for your lips but also has a tint to add some colour. Make sure they're ultra-moisturizing and contain SPF.

The mood is… Warm…Diaphanous…Iridescent…Dewy…Delicate…Sunkissed…Radiant…Fresh

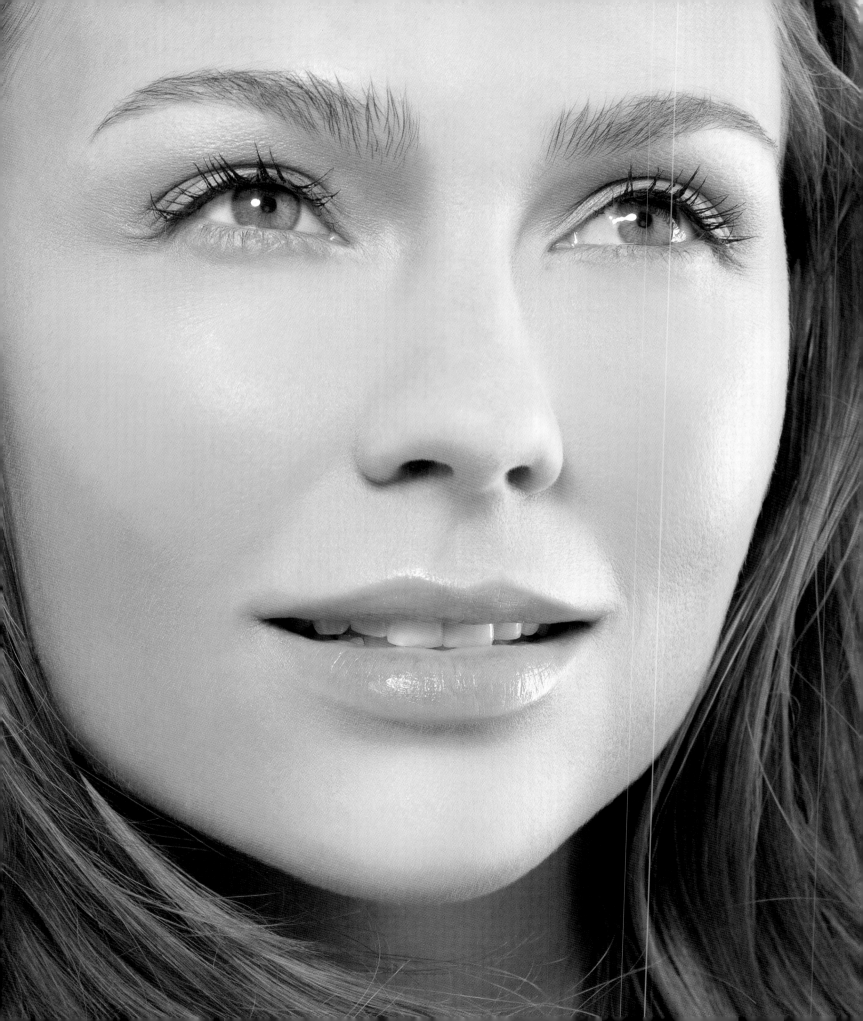

Spring/summer glow

Sometimes it feels as if winter will never end and skin will stay pale for ever. Here's how to add some glow.

» Use radiance crème under foundation. This is more subtle than when you dab it on top as a highlighter.

» Olive and golden skins tend to look sallow by this time of the year. Instead of using a gold-coloured foundation or bronzer, which will accentuate the yellow, apply a plum or berry blush to counteract it.

» Don't try to cover very pale skin with a darker foundation – match to your natural skin tone and add colour with blush. Peach tones give a sunkissed radiance to the skin.

Inspiration for spring/summer looks

The arrival of spring heralds the use of lighter, brighter colours for garden-fresh looks to go with the season.

Bold colours for eyes

Create a wash of colour across the eye with pale leaf greens, daffodil yellow and crocus lilac, or use soft, clear shades to provide an accent of colour at the lash line against a neutral peachy beige. Try unusual colour combinations, but keep lips soft and neutral with a rose or peach gloss or stain.

1 If eyes are red, blend a dot of foundation or concealer over the lid. To prevent creasing, brush a natural colour powder across the lid to absorb any oil.

2 Use a small eye brush with dense natural hairs. Load the brush with powder, tapping away any excess. Begin by applying at the root of the lash, pushing the powder in, rather than stroking it across the lid.

3 Use a slightly larger brush to blend the colour up to the socket line and a little way beyond, creating a soft edge at the outer corner of the eye. Don't apply colour at the socket, since this will mean blending it too far above.

4 To increase the colour intensity, apply more colour at the lash line and blend up.

5 Add a sweep of highlighter under the browbone and keep the look simple with a lash tint or clear mascara.

DAY TO NIGHT Add a sweep of metallic eyeliner in pewter, green or peacock blue, and define the lashes with volumizing mascara.

My secret Use a little white eyeshadow to highlight the inner corner of the eye to make your eyes sparkle and pop.

Spring pastels

Pale greys or silver are easy to wear, while pastel spring-flower colours – lilac, yellow or green – give a fresh, innocent look.

EYES For day a simple wash of colour over the eye is brightening, but for evening try using the same pastel colours for a smoky eye. For example, highlight with a very light lilac and use a soft purple on the root of the lash. A touch of smudged liner in a matching shade – perhaps even peacock blue – gives a look that's fresh but strong. Curl the lashes to frame the eyes, then use a lash tint to darken and separate the lashes.

FACE Luminous is the buzzword of the season, so prepare your face properly. Then use a light foundation, mousse or tinted moisturizer. If your complexion is good, just use all-over radiance crème and for evening add illuminator on cheekbones and browbones.

CHEEKS Use a tint or crème blush in a natural fresh pink, so that your cheeks look as though you've pinched them – use very little product to start with and build up the colour gradually.

LIPS Rosebud lips are natural, full and bee-stung. First moisturize with a gently plumping lip balm. Many of the tints and stains for cheeks work beautifully on lips, too. Add either a light, almost neutral gloss over the top or a pinker one for more colour. A gloss that is silky rather than glossy will give a subtler sheen.

DAY TO NIGHT Dress up this very natural make-up by increasing the shimmer or adding a metallic eyeliner.

Summer nights

For long summer evenings, make-up should be simple but feminine with a soft, flattering golden glow.

EYES A sweep of warm orange bronze right across the lid and blended out past the socket line makes the perfect summery evening look for all skin tones. Use a golden highlighter under the browbone and a deeper brown on the lash line. Use an eyeliner brush to push colour in at the root of the lashes, extending it a little at the corner. If you prefer, begin with a pencil liner to define the eye by thickening the upper lash line and then go over it with the powder. For a more daring look, use contrasting purple or berry-coloured eyeliner. Then apply black volumizing mascara.

FACE Use plenty of moisturizer to make skin luminous. If you have an even complexion, just use a radiance crème and touches of concealer around the nose and under the eyes. If not, either use a tinted moisturizer that matches your skin, or blend a liquid foundation on cheeks and nose. When this has soaked in, add a radiance product for a dewy glow – crème or liquid is perfect, as you can really work it into the skin. If you're tanned, blend a little golden highlighter on cheekbones, under the browbone and on the forehead.

CHEEKS Soft pink or warm apricot are flattering in summer light. Either dab colour on the apple of the cheeks and blend a little way along the cheekbones, or apply a touch of blush in the triangle under the cheekbone to help shape the face subtly and don't add any colour on the apple or the cheekbone itself.

LIPS Line and fill in the lips with a natural pink pencil to give a full, even shape. Finish with a soft sheen gloss or a slick of balm.

My secret A touch of loose shimmer powder on the middle of the lids draws attention to your eyes.

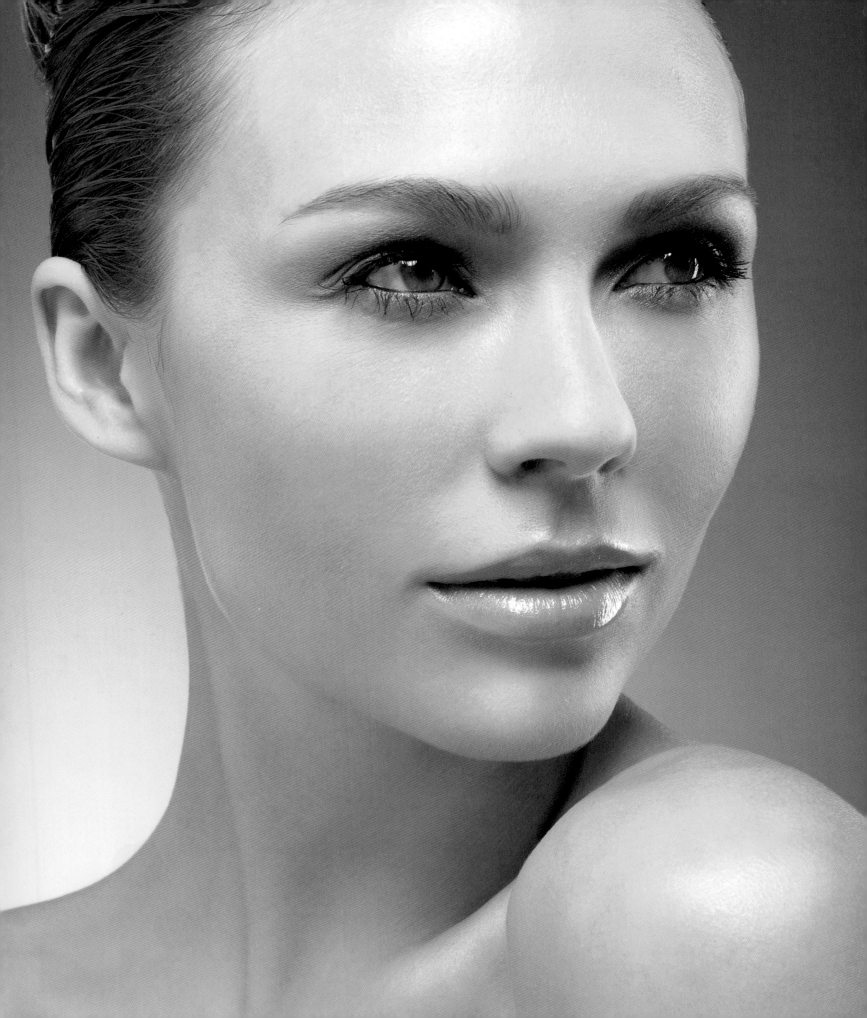

autumn/winter

Cold weather is harsh on skin and central heating dries it out. We wrap up in coats, scarves and gloves, but leave our faces exposed, and while wearing a balaclava isn't the solution, skin does need extra protection at this time of year to avoid getting rough, chapped or red. Here is my advice to keep it at its best.

Protection and hydration

Start exfoliating every other day to prevent any flaky areas from forming, and use a more intensive moisturizer to protect the skin. Look for rich oil-based balms with SPF and vitamin K to counteract redness. Pat it into cleansed skin and let it sink in before you put on make-up.

Moisturizing make-up

FACE Consider switching to a heavier-coverage foundation – on thoroughly moisturized skin a crème foundation won't cake or look too thick. Apply it sparingly with fingers or a sponge and work it into the skin thoroughly. Your skin will probably get paler, and you should change your foundation or concealer to reflect that. Invest in an illuminating base to use underneath your foundation to give winter skin instant luminosity. Avoid using too much powder, which can be drying – an overly matte look is easily spoiled in the rain.

QUICK FIX In a centrally heated environment, keep a water spritzer to hand to refresh skin and make-up during the day.

EYES Eyebrows should be strong to provide a confident frame for the face, so consider having yours shaped professionally at the start of the season and invest in a brow kit to keep them tidy and defined.

Eyes often water in the cold and wind, so avoid eyeliner or mascara that is likely to run. I'm a huge fan of natural beauty in summer, but I like bringing in richer colours in autumn. Jewel and berry colours are fantastic for eyeshadow – try the brighter tones in a moisturizing crème shadow on the lid or to define the socket, as well as the smoky shades that look so sexy. Avoid too much pink, as this brings out redness in the eyes and skin. Shimmery metallic eyeshadow is great for winter drama.

CHEEKS Put bronzer away – the sunkissed all-over shimmer of spring/summer should be replaced with matte, nude colours. Buy a matte blush a shade or two darker than your natural colour. Cool blue-based pinks give a wintry flush. If your skin is very dry, crème blush will be more moisturizing than powder.

LIPS Carry a wax balm and reapply frequently. Look for a lipgloss with moisturizers or vitamin E to protect the lips while adding shine. Treat yourself to a flattering red lipstick, preferably matte rather than gloss, so it is less easy to smudge. Define the lips with liner in a matching shade before applying the lipstick using a brush.

QUICK FIX A stain is perfect for those who want just a wash of red on their lips rather than a full-on red pout.

The mood is…Seductive…Strong…Intense…Deep…Defined…Rich…Jewel colours…Smouldering

Autumn/winter glow

If skin is ultra-dry or chapped, foundation will look flaky and unattractive.

» Make sure your cleanser is non-drying – crèmes and oils are kinder than alcohol-based wipes for removing make-up, and water-based cleanser should be non-soap-based. Use an exfoliator twice a week to remove any dead skin.

» Increase your hydration. Use a few drops of a facial oil underneath your daily moisturizer and massage in an especially rich cream at night.

» Primers create a great base for foundations to glide onto the skin and help to keep them in place all day.

» Try a foundation with a pink or pearlescent sheen and add radiance crème or highlighter. Use a dab of creamy peach or pink blush for a naturally flushed cheek.

Inspiration for autumn/winter looks

As the light fashions of summer are replaced by the structured silhouettes of winter, a stronger make-up expression seems more fitting, with the emphasis on boldly defined eyes and intense lip colours. When the nights draw in, smouldering eyes are more appealing, and foundation becomes less dewy, with richer hydrating formulations that keep moisture loss to a minimum.

Bold brows

Strong brows frame the face and create drama; they also balance out strong lips. Brush brows upwards and emphasize the shape with a brow pencil or an eyeshadow one or two shades darker than your natural colour, elongating them slightly towards the outer corners. For a more dramatic look, make them squared and sharpened, bold and pencilled in.

Reinventing summer's vibrant eye colours

In winter bright colours – especially blues and greens – can be applied across the whole eyelid and teamed with graphic black eyeliner for a clean, modern look.

1 Use a primer across your lids to smooth the texture and even out any redness.

2 Sweep colour across the lids with a brush, taking it up to the socket line. Apply dry for a sheer wash of colour, or wet for a bolder result.

3 Outline the whole of the eyes, including the inner rims, with black eyeliner.

4 Wear a nude shade on the lips to balance the look.

5 Keep the complexion muted – all you need is a sheer tawny powder blush swept lightly across the cheeks.

My secret Treat dull skin to a mask and stimulate the circulation by giving yourself a facial massage.

Smoky eyes

In the cooler months smoky eyes come into their own. Choose two dark shades and blend them together, using a smudging brush for the best effect. Line the inner rims and highlight the corners and browbones with a lighter shadow, such as silver (see pages 98–9). Using glitter, shimmer and metallics is a fun, eye-catching take on this classic look, while vivid colours with false lashes and bold eyeliner create extra drama. Try colours such as burnished gold, silver, jade or midnight blue.

Sexy cat eyes

This look smoulders in the winter months. Use black eyeliner, or purple if you're fair. Starting at the inner corners, draw the liner all the way along your upper lash line, then flick it up and out at the end. Take a taupe eyeshadow across the browbone and blend it well. Curl the lashes, then apply two coats of lengthening mascara. For extra impact, apply individual false lashes at the outer edges of the eyes.

Red lips

With a shade to suit all complexions, red lips look chic and timeless (see pages 132–3). If you have fair hair and skin with pink tones, cooler reds will look best. Mediterranean and olive skins suit orange-based reds and rich cherry red. Dark skin looks beautiful in deeper burgundy reds.

My secret Keep the focus on one aspect – eyes or lips. The rest of your look should be natural, with velvety matte foundation and a little light blush – no shimmery bronzers.

WINTER SKIN – PROBLEMS AND SOLUTIONS

CHAPPED LIPS Lips don't produce their own oil, so they tend to dry out and crack. *Avoid lip balms that contain mineral oil or glycerine – although these feel silky, they actually leave lips drier. Look for balms containing beeswax or shea butter.*

DRY FLAKY SKIN Temperature extremes deprive the skin of moisture. This slows down the renewal process – the shedding of dead skin cells to make way for new skin – leaving a dry, flaky surface. *Gently exfoliate twice a week or even every other day, and use a good moisturizer.*

RED SKIN Pale, sensitive skin can suffer from redness. Icy winds weaken the moisture barrier, leaving skin prone to inflammation. *Keep skin hydrated and protected with gentle cleansers and SPF moisturizer. A targeted anti-redness cream will help to rebuild the barrier and soothe.*

RED EYES Wind-induced tears make mascara run and can leave the eye area red and irritated. *Wear waterproof mascara and apply a little concealer or a yellow-tinted eye base over your lids and at the corners of the eyes to neutralize redness.*

BRITTLE NAILS Central heating and winter weather dry out nails, making them brittle and prone to flaking. *Massage almond oil into the nails and cuticles every night, and use a moisturizing hand cream. If you wear nail polish, use a conditioning base coat to protect the nail bed.*

LINES AND WRINKLES Skin needs moisture to look plump and line-free, so the drying effects of cold weather mean that fine lines and wrinkles become more visible. *For an intensive moisture boost, apply a hydrating serum underneath your moisturizer.*

TOP TEN MUST-HAVES FOR YOUR MAKE-UP BAG

LOOSE POWDER – THIS REMOVES EXCESS OIL FROM THE SKIN AND GIVES A VELVETY FINISH. LIGHTLY DUST OVER THE FACE, PAYING SPECIAL ATTENTION TO AREAS PRONE TO OILINESS, SUCH AS THE CHIN, FOREHEAD AND TIP OF THE NOSE. IF YOUR SKIN IS VERY DRY, THERE IS NO NEED TO APPLY POWDER.

LASH CURLERS – CURLING THE LASHES IS CRUCIAL FOR ACCENTUATING THE EYES. START AS CLOSE TO THE ROOT AS POSSIBLE AND CURL TWO TO THREE TIMES, EACH TIME MOVING THE CURLERS A FEW MILLIMETRES UP THE LASHES.

PRIMER – THIS ACTS AS AN UNDERCOAT, PROVIDING A BASE FOR FOUNDATION AND MAKING SURE IT LASTS LONGER.

TWEEZERS – WELL-GROOMED BROWS FRAME THE FACE AND GIVE YOUR LOOK A SOPHISTICATED POLISH. TWEEZE ANY STRAY HAIRS EARLY IN THE DAY TO ALLOW ANY REDNESS TO FADE.

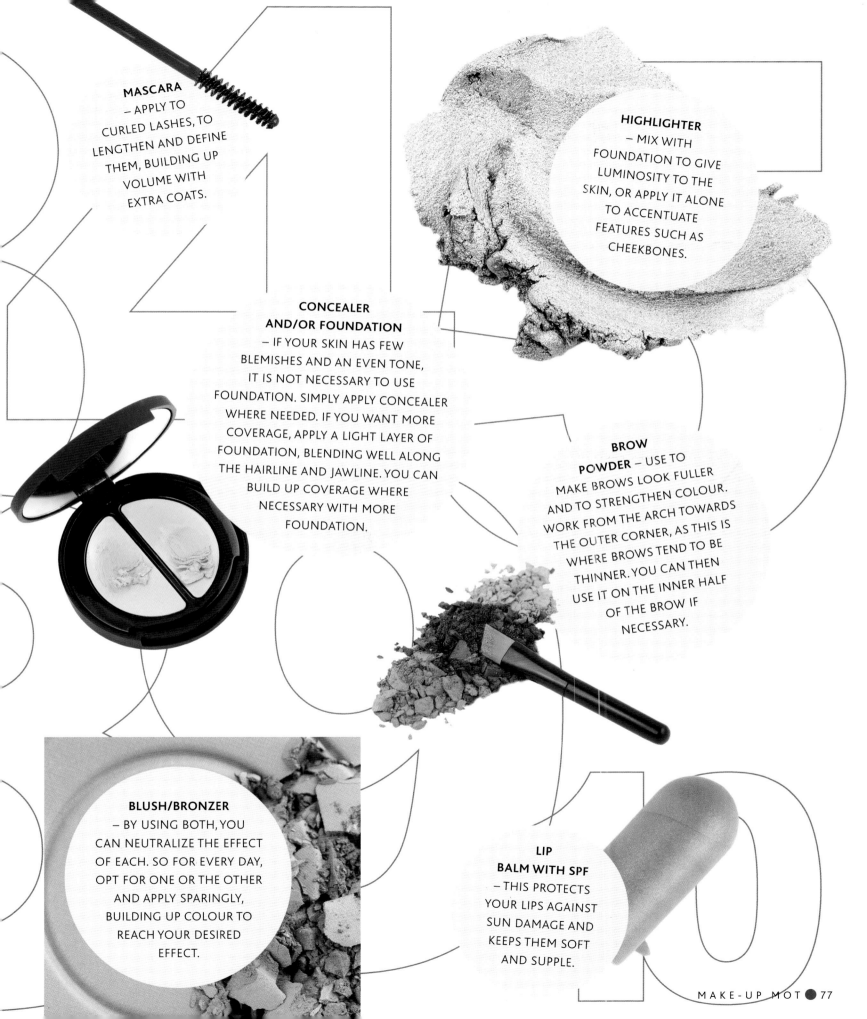

MASCARA
– APPLY TO CURLED LASHES, TO LENGTHEN AND DEFINE THEM, BUILDING UP VOLUME WITH EXTRA COATS.

HIGHLIGHTER
– MIX WITH FOUNDATION TO GIVE LUMINOSITY TO THE SKIN, OR APPLY IT ALONE TO ACCENTUATE FEATURES SUCH AS CHEEKBONES.

CONCEALER AND/OR FOUNDATION
– IF YOUR SKIN HAS FEW BLEMISHES AND AN EVEN TONE, IT IS NOT NECESSARY TO USE FOUNDATION. SIMPLY APPLY CONCEALER WHERE NEEDED. IF YOU WANT MORE COVERAGE, APPLY A LIGHT LAYER OF FOUNDATION, BLENDING WELL ALONG THE HAIRLINE AND JAWLINE. YOU CAN BUILD UP COVERAGE WHERE NECESSARY WITH MORE FOUNDATION.

BROW POWDER
– USE TO MAKE BROWS LOOK FULLER AND TO STRENGTHEN COLOUR. WORK FROM THE ARCH TOWARDS THE OUTER CORNER, AS THIS IS WHERE BROWS TEND TO BE THINNER. YOU CAN THEN USE IT ON THE INNER HALF OF THE BROW IF NECESSARY.

BLUSH/BRONZER
– BY USING BOTH, YOU CAN NEUTRALIZE THE EFFECT OF EACH. SO FOR EVERY DAY, OPT FOR ONE OR THE OTHER AND APPLY SPARINGLY, BUILDING UP COLOUR TO REACH YOUR DESIRED EFFECT.

LIP BALM WITH SPF
– THIS PROTECTS YOUR LIPS AGAINST SUN DAMAGE AND KEEPS THEM SOFT AND SUPPLE.

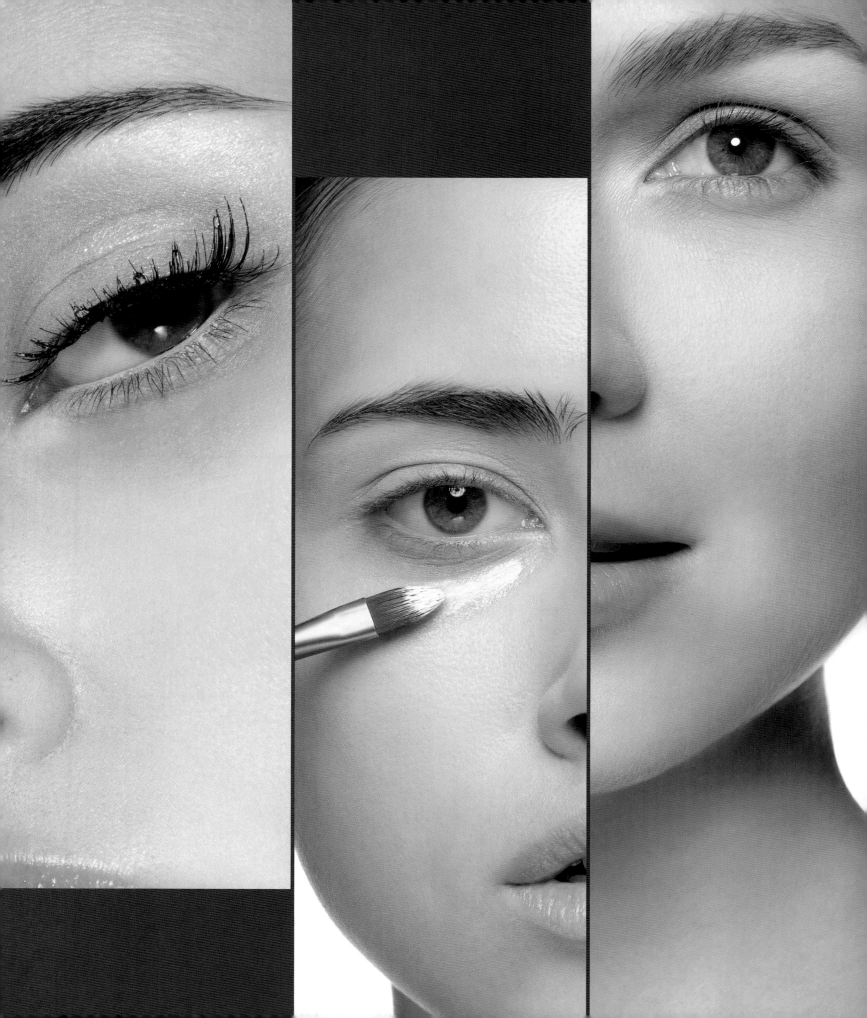

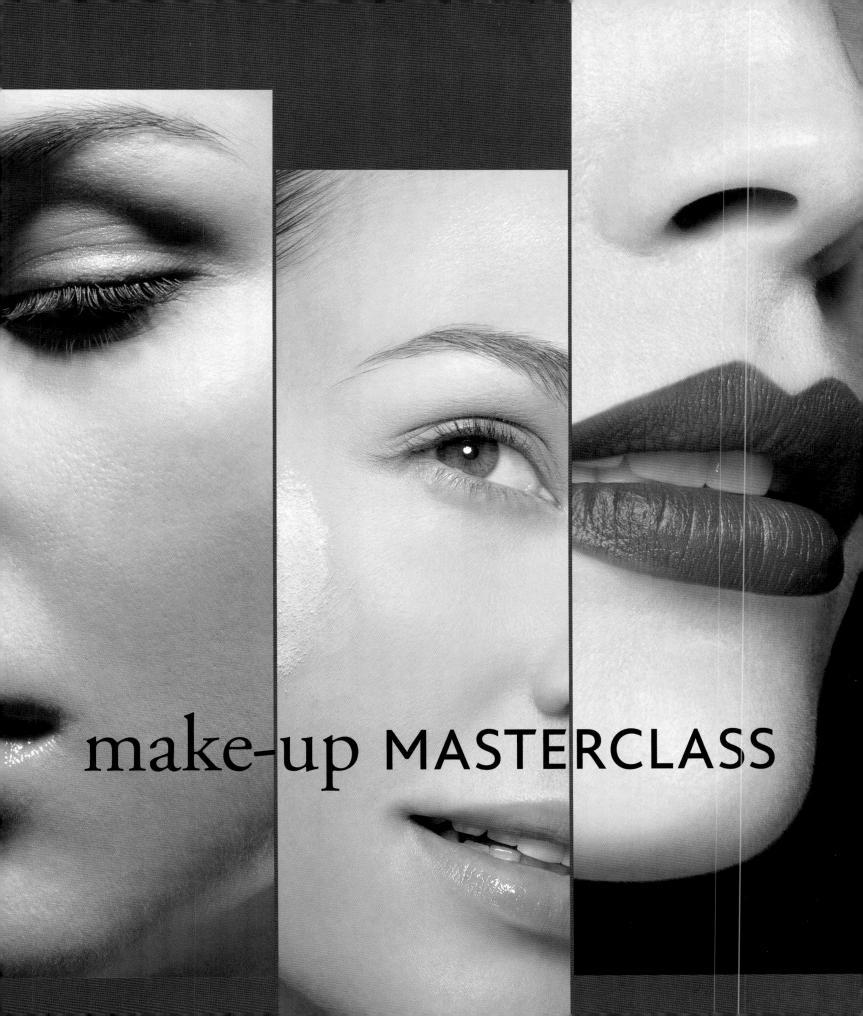

make-up MASTERCLASS

MAKING UP YOUR FACE

Applying make-up is a very personal thing – every woman I know has a routine that they tend to follow – and while there are no real rights and wrongs, the following tips will help you to achieve the most professional results.

How you apply make-up should be dictated by the look you're creating. If you're going for dramatic eye make-up, prep the skin and make up your eyes before doing your face. If flecks of eyeshadow or mascara drop on the face, you can remove them without ruining the rest of your make-up. If you're creating a natural look with minimal eye make-up, you can focus on the face first, ensuring a flawless, radiant complexion.

The order in which you should work also depends on the formulations you use – all crème finishes need to be applied before setting make-up with powder, otherwise they won't blend smoothly. Powder blush needs to be applied after powder, or it will stick to foundation and give a patchy finish.

Ten steps to perfect make-up

1 Start with clean, bare skin.

2 Use a moisturizer with SPF on the face and décolletage.

3 Use an eye cream to hydrate the eye area.

4 Apply a primer, if you wish.

5 If you are creating dramatic eyes, apply your eye make-up now, before you do your face.

6 Apply foundation where desired, blending it well around the hairline and jawbone.

7 Use concealer where needed, such as under the eyes, around the nostrils and on any blemishes.

8 If you are wearing a crème blush or cheek stain, apply it now, blending well.

9 Apply a light sheer powder to set the foundation and remove shine. If you prefer powder blush, apply it now.

10 Do your lips last, to avoid smudging. Use a touch of make-up remover on a cotton bud to correct mistakes.

Creating balance

One of the core principles of make-up artistry is that every make-up look is based on one of four eye/lip combinations (see opposite). This is about creating balance, and trial and error will determine which combination is the most flattering for your features.

» **Light eyes/light lips** *(top left)* A nude 'no make-up' look, which is all about creating radiant skin with eyes and lips softly defined in a subtle neutral palette – perfect everyday make-up.

» **Light eyes/dark lips** *(top right)* A vintage look that works well if your mouth is your best feature. Keep eyes neutral and bring all the focus to the mouth with luscious red, pink or brown lipstick.

» **Dark eyes/light lips** *(bottom left)* A classic sexy but sophisticated night-time look, with smouldering defined eyes in smoky colours paired with understated lips.

» **Dark eyes/dark lips** *(bottom right)* This is the full monty of a look and spells serious high-maintenance glamour – perfect for a special occasion.

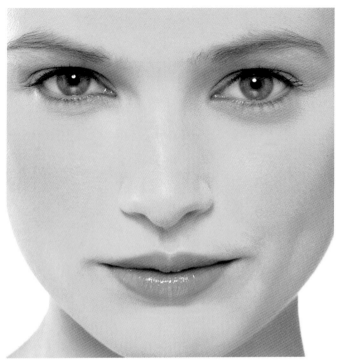
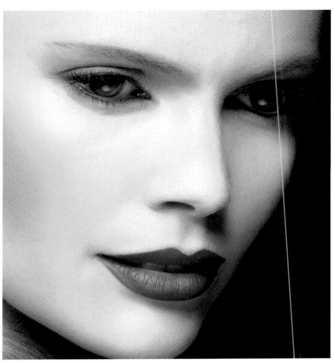
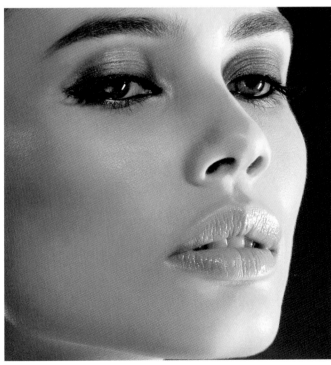
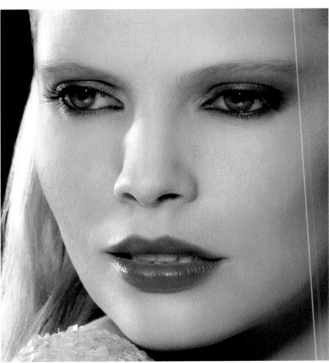

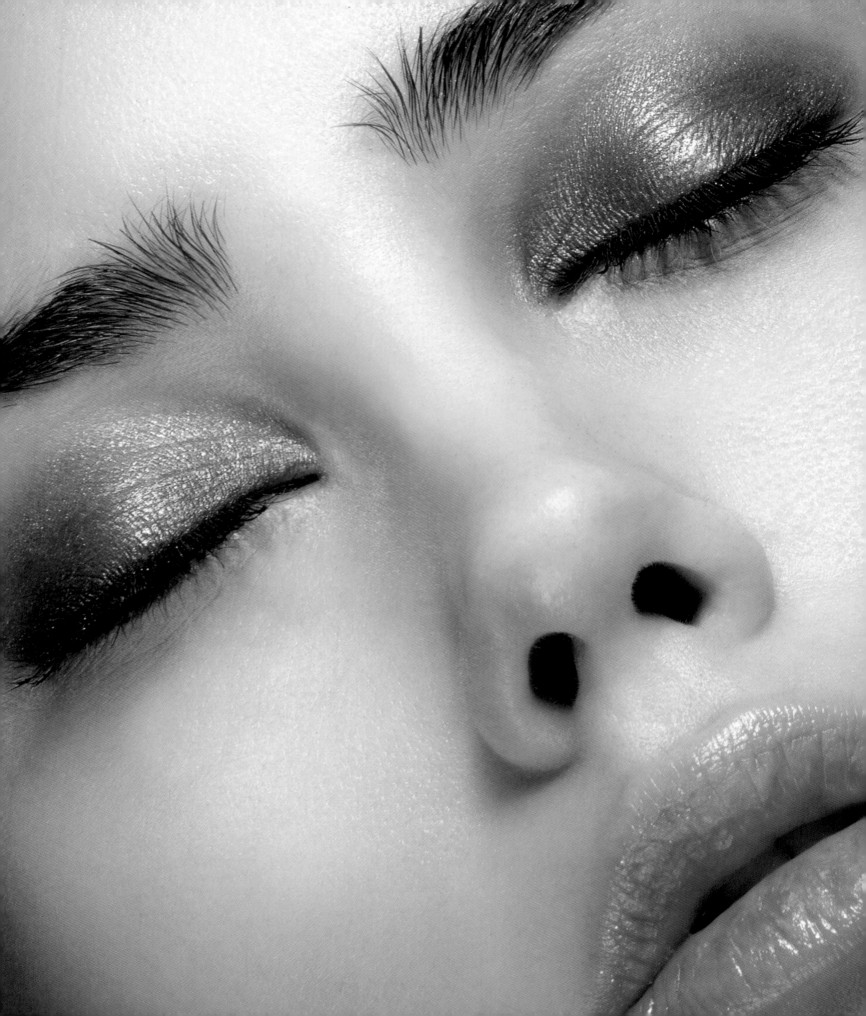

EXQUISITE EYES

Our eyes express our emotions and betray our thoughts, glinting when we're angry, pooling with tears when we're sad and sparkling with happiness when we laugh.

Eye make-up can reveal a lot about our personality – or the persona we wish to portray at any given time. It can transform us from capable business woman to sexy siren, from natural and pretty to sultry and glamorous in an instant. It's a wonderful tool that allows us to express different sides of our personality. Like all make-up, it should boost our confidence, enhance and flatter, enabling our true self to shine at its very best. Experiment with different looks and have fun playing with colour and texture.

Look after your eyes

The skin around the eyes is much thinner than on the rest of the face and signs of ageing will show there first. Stress, tiredness, overexposure to the sun and poor diet all take their toll. Try not to strain your eyes by reading in poor light, watching too much television or staring at your computer for too long. Wear sunglasses in bright weather to protect the eyes and prevent squinting. Do your best to have a good night's sleep and eat a healthy diet.

My secret To combat dark undereye circles, dab a tiny amount of creamy white eyeshadow in the inner corners of the eyelids, top and bottom. If your skin is dark, use a light brown shade. Blend well, then apply concealer on top and around the eyes.

eye shapes

The shape of your eyes, how they are set and the size of your eyelids all influence the way you should make up your eyes for the most flattering effect. Understanding a few basic principles will help you to make the most of your eyes.

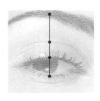

EYELID PROPORTIONS

The eyes on the left illustrate different eyelid proportions. The top eye has a deeper space between the browbone and socket crease and a larger visible lid, making it ideal for heavy eyeliner. Most looks are easy to achieve on this type of eye, but the socket crease may need definition. The bottom eye has a heavy lid, so darkening and thickening the socket crease gives the impression it is higher, opening up the eye. Keep highlighter just under the browbone.

TOP TIP

To highlight an area to make it stand out, use a light colour; to make it recede or to minimize it, use a dark colour.

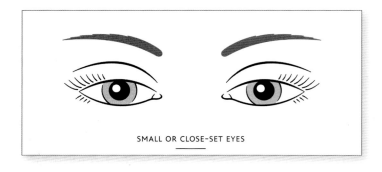

SMALL OR CLOSE-SET EYES

Small or close-set eyes

The average space between a pair of eyes is approximately the width of one eye. If your eyes are closer than this, you have close-set eyes. To create the illusion that the eyes are farther apart apply a light colour to the inner corner of your eyes and three-quarters of the way across your lid. Apply a darker colour to the outer corner of your eyes and blend it outwards to 'stretch' the eye. Highlight under the browbone and in the inner corners. Apply eyeliner to the outer corner of the top and bottom lids only and smudge inwards to soften. Open up your eyes and create the illusion of larger eyes by applying beige or white eyeliner around the inner rims.

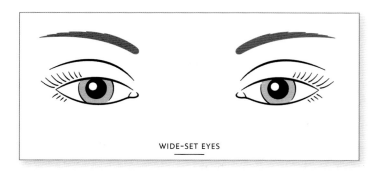

WIDE-SET EYES

Wide-set eyes

If the space between your eyes is wider than the width of one eye, your eyes will be considered wide set. To create the illusion that the eyes are slightly closer together apply a dark colour at the inner corner of your eyes and blend a lighter shade towards the outer corner. Emphasize the socket line with a dark colour near the inner corner, fading as you reach the outer corner – don't take it beyond. Mascara should be thicker on the lashes at the inner corner of the eye to draw the focus inwards.

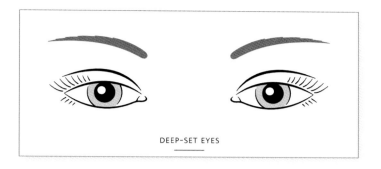

DEEP-SET EYES

Deep-set eyes

Deep-set eyes appear slightly sunken into the socket and have a prominent browbone. To bring the eyes forward to make them more noticeable apply highlighter over the lid to just above the hollow. Blend a mid shade into the socket line, then blend highlighter under the browbone. Draw a fine line of eyeliner along the upper lash line.

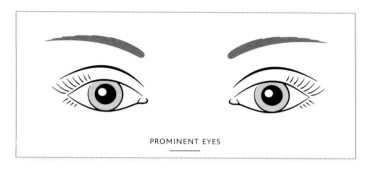

PROMINENT EYES

Prominent eyes

If your eyelids and eyes tend to protrude from your face, you have prominent eyes. To make the lid recede blend a dark colour onto the lid and just under the bottom lashes at the outer corner of the eye. Blend highlighter just under the browbone. Draw eyeliner along the top lashes and use a brush to blend it well into the dark eyeshadow.

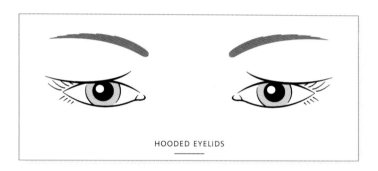

HOODED EYELIDS

Hooded eyelids

If your eyelids appear slightly closed, they are considered hooded. To make the eyes appear larger and more open, minimize the fleshy part of the lid. Apply a highlighter colour to the entire eye area. Blend a darker shade from the base of the upper lash line over your entire eye socket – this will help it to recede. Sweep the darker colour underneath your lower lash line for definition. Hooded eyes look fabulous with a well-defined upper and lower lash line.

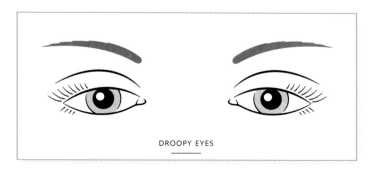

DROOPY EYES

Droopy eyes

'Puppy-dog' eyes that slope downwards at the outer corners can make the face look sad. Create lift at the outer corners to give the face a brighter expression. Blend a mid colour over the lid and up to the brow. Apply a darker colour to the socket line, raising it at the outer corner. Blend a highlighter at the outer corner of the eye. Draw eyeliner from the centre of the upper lash line to the outer corner and smudge, blending the colour slightly upwards – this acts like a flick to elongate and lift the eye. You can wear colour on the lower lash line, but stop just in from the outer corner of your eyes. When you apply mascara, concentrate on the middle of your lashes – defining lashes at the outer corners will accentuate droopiness.

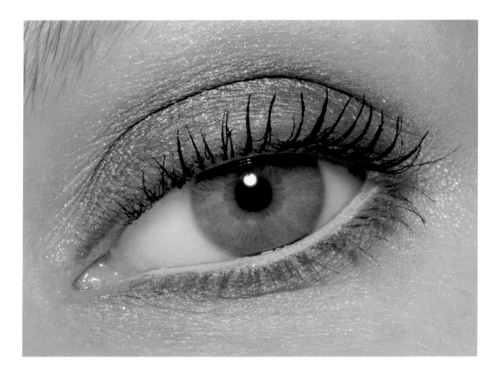

Orange is opposite blue on the artist's colour wheel, so eyeshadow with orange tones, such as shimmery copper, will make blue eyes 'pop'.

colour

Neutral shades of beige and brown have their place, but with all the juicy colours available, you don't want to play it so safe that you stick to just one palette. Here are some pointers to help you to experiment without looking like a teenager on your way to the disco.

Adding colour

It's best to use no more than two or three hues. Here are three simple ways to add colour:

» Create a neutral eye with a pale shade under the browbone and a mid colour on the lid blended to just above the socket. Try a bright shade along the lash line.

» Apply a wash of colour – pastels and juicy shades work well – over the whole lid, blending a little way out and over the socket line at the outer corners.

» If you're happy with the way you apply eyeshadow, try the same style but in a different colour palette. For example, instead of chocolate on the lash line and in the socket, try deep purple and highlight with lilac-tinted white instead of cream.

The theory

Rules are there to be broken, but there is a science behind choosing colours for your eye make-up according to the colour of your eyes. It works on the same principle as an artist's colour wheel. Any three colours next to each other on a 12-colour wheel are related colours, while colours directly opposite each other are complementary.

To enhance and exaggerate your eye colour, choose a palette of related colours – flooding the area around the iris with similar shades will intensify its colour. Conversely, to make your eye colour 'pop' with dramatic colour contrast, choose a palette of complementary colours.

» Line blue eyes with golden brown or a shade of grey that's lighter than your eyes.

» Line green eyes with copper or auburn, or be more daring with red or orange.

» Line brown eyes with mossy green to make them smoulder.

» Line hazel eyes with deep sapphire or violet.

Blue eyes
Enhance by selecting an eyeshadow in a complementary colour to the iris. The complementary colour to blue is orange, so shadows with an ochre, copper or terracotta tone create a complementary contrast. Peach has a tint of orange, so is a perfect shade for a subtle daytime look. Opting for a dark blue eyeshadow will enhance blue eyes by surrounding the iris with an intense depth of colour.

Green eyes
Green eyes can be set off by selecting an eyeshadow in a complementary colour to the iris. The complementary colour to green is technically red, so eyeshadows with a red, violet, wine, burgundy or maroon tone will create a complementary contrast. Pink is a tint of red, so would be a perfect shade for the daytime.

Brown eyes
Brown does not have a complementary colour, but most eyeshadow colours suit brown eyes. To intensify the colour of the iris, opt for shades of brown, such as chocolate, soft browns and taupes. Purples and greens, particularly pistachio green, look great on brown eyes, while light pastel shades also work very well.

Hazel eyes
As hazel eyes have flecks of gold, brown and green, the complementary colours are tones of blue, violet, purple and red. To enhance the colour of your eyes, opt for olive and emerald greens, gold and orange tones. A blue eyeshadow will emphasize any blue skin tones, such as those in dark undereye circles. Make sure your skin looks flawless and you have covered any blemishes.

Neutrals
Neutral colours – creams, beiges, taupes and browns – can be worn to great effect, whatever your eye colour. Warm neutrals, which contain more yellow pigment, are suited to warm brown, green and hazel eyes, while cool neutrals, containing more blue pigment, are best suited to deep brown, blue, grey, cool green and cool hazel eyes.

TOP TIP
Test colours on your hand before you buy. Some eyeshadows look fantastic in the palette but produce such a light wash on the eye that it is hard to build up intensity. Some colours that look bright in the palette are much softer on the skin.

beautiful brows

Well-shaped eyebrows can make a real difference to your look and take years off. They frame the face, open it up and give the eyes definition. Some of the most famous signature looks of film stars have been a lot to do with their eyebrows – think of Audrey Hepburn and Elizabeth Taylor. Most people need do little more than keep their eyebrows tidy and groomed, emphasizing the natural arch, but more adventurous reshaping can have a dramatic effect. Draw on different shapes to experiment with what suits you, or have your eyebrows shaped professionally by a brow specialist and maintain the shape yourself.

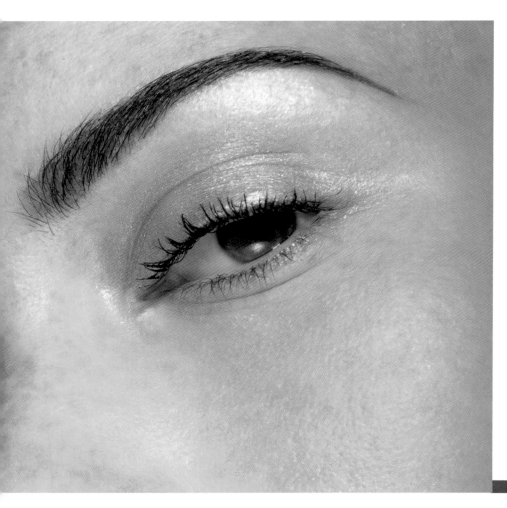

The classic shape

Finding the brow shape that suits you is not difficult – your brow probably already arches in the right place and just needs tidying. The most common shape is slightly squared off at the nose with an arch two thirds of the way along and a tapered end. Here are some guidelines:

» Brows should begin in line with the inner corner of the eyes and be a full eye-width apart.

» The highest point of the arch should fall above the outer edge of your iris.

» Hold a brush or pencil in front of your nose and tilt it diagonally to the outer corner of your eye. Follow the same line up until it meets the brow to find the outer point. Depending on your brows, you may want to extend them up to this point with a brow pencil (see opposite) or pluck any stray hairs.

TIPS AND HINTS FOR BROWS

» Set the eyebrows by spritzing hairspray onto a brow brush before combing. Or try a slick of hair gel or clear mascara.

» Brows are emphasized not only by darkening the brow itself, but also by highlighting under the brow using a pale colour to define the line.

» Eyebrows can draw attention away from droopy eyes. If the brow slopes gently away, continuing in a line just beyond the corner, it lifts the entire eye.

» If you change your hair colour, you may also need to gently bleach your eyebrows to match.

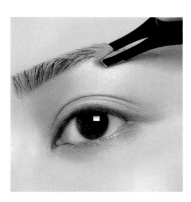

» Pluck hairs one by one, a line at a time, making sure each root is in the area you want to pluck. Start at the side of your brow nearest your nose and work outwards. Pluck below the brow line, removing all the hairs in the lid/socket area. Any obvious stray hairs above the brow can be plucked, but generally it's better to trim or bleach hairs above the brow line rather than pluck whole lines, as this thins the brows.

» Brush the eyebrow hairs so they lie flat or slightly upwards to reveal any others that need neatening, and trim any stray long hairs with nail scissors.

Shaping techniques

Professional techniques include waxing and threading. Threading originated in Asia and is an accurate, fast and less messy way of removing unwanted hair with nothing more than a tensioned thread. Electrolysis requires a course of treatments and can be painful, but the results are permanent. For DIY shaping, plucking is the best option.

Tools

Angled tweezers, white pencil, eyebrow brush and comb, nail scissors, angled stiff brush and powder or eyebrow pencil.

Trimming

» Brush the eyebrow hairs upwards with a brow comb and trim any hairs over the top line of the brow with nail scissors.

» Brush the hairs down and trim again if necessary.

» Brush the brow back into shape. You can now see the hairs that need to be plucked.

Plucking and tweezing

» Pluck after showering when pores are open and the hair is softer, or open the pores with a hot flannel. Make sure your face is free of make-up and moisturizer, so the tweezers don't slip.

» Dip a small flat angled brush into some brow powder, then with upward strokes sketch in your ideal brow. Use a white pencil to colour under the lower line of the shape you want, making sure both sides are even – the hairs you've drawn over are the ones to pluck. I prefer to draw my ideal shape in this way instead of using a mass-produced stencil.

» Only pluck in good light. Always pull in the direction in which the hair is growing. It is less painful and the hair is less likely to break.

Defining and colouring

» Eyebrow pencils and powder can fill in any gaps. I like to use a pencil to extend the brow at the outer corner, and powder with an angled brush to fill any gaps or to define the arch.

» Never use a brow pencil in a solid line like an eyeliner. To create the illusion of fine hairs, use short feathery irregular-length strokes that follow the pattern of hair growth: at the inner corner this is angled upwards, from the arch onwards, horizontal or down.

» Brow powder is better than eyeshadow, as it is matte with no shimmer and less creamy, giving a less solid look. Apply using a firm angled brush with short feathery strokes in the same direction as hairs are growing. Define the arch, drawing just inside the last couple of hairs for a natural look. Some brow kits also come with wax to help 'set' the powder.

» The colour should complement your hair colour, but choose a shade lighter for a natural look or exactly the same shade for a more dramatic effect. Brunettes can use any shade of dark brown; blondes should look for soft browns or taupe; redheads should go for taupe, chestnut or auburn; if you have black hair, use very dark brown or deep charcoal – black tends to be too heavy.

a fine line

Eyeliner can be dramatic or subtle, sexy or innocent. Different textures can be applied in different ways to accessorize the eyes – from liquid and gel to pencil, in coloured, glitter or metallic finishes. Eyeliner can be drawn all the way around the eye or just along the top or bottom; you can draw halfway along or create flicks that extend beyond the eye; make the line strong and defined or soft and smudged; draw on the inner rim or on the outside of the lashes – anything goes. Pencil is the easiest eyeliner to master and the most forgiving, producing a blunt line that can be smudged. Liquid liner creates a precise line for a super-glam look, but calls for a steady hand. Gel liner, which comes in many colours, gives a similar effect, but is easier to apply.

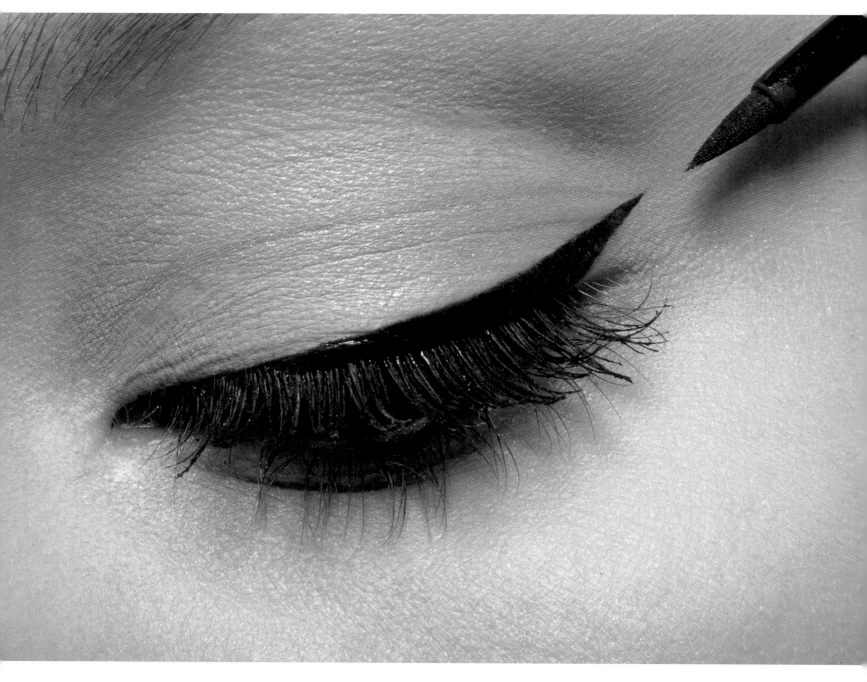

Opposite Gel liner is fast-drying, waterproof and long-lasting. The pen applicator makes it easier to achieve a precise line along the upper lashes with a flick at the outer corner.

Top right For high-maintenance glamour, liquid liner is applied with a fine brush and a steady hand.

Centre and bottom right Pencil liner is very versatile, giving a blunt line that can be smudged with a special tool for a soft, smoky look.

Applying gel and liquid eyeliner

» If using a pen applicator, hold it at an angle, pointing slightly downwards and use a light hand – pressing gives an overly thick line.

» If using a brush, choose a fine, dense brush and clean it thoroughly after every use.

» Rest your elbow on the table to steady your hand.

» Hold your eyelid taut to eliminate any creases.

» If you have deep-set eyes or heavy lids, keep your eyes closed until the liner is dry.

» Use an oil-based eye make-up remover to correct any slips.

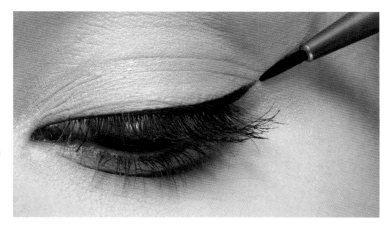

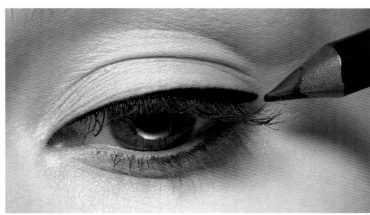

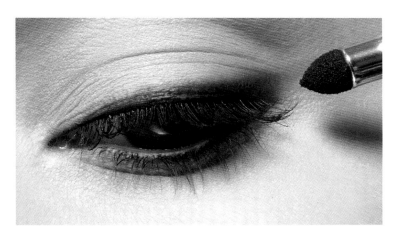

Applying pencil eyeliner

» Choose a soft, creamy pencil that will glide on without dragging the skin.

» Sharpen the pencil, but not to a dagger point.

» The most common mistake is to draw eyeliner too high, leaving a noticeable strip of skin between the lashes and the liner. To avoid this, work the pencil tip right in at the root of the lash. Start just in from the outer corner and draw along the lash line towards the mid point. Use short feathery strokes or draw a series of dots and smudge them together. As you gain confidence, draw a solid line for precise definition.

» As you pass the mid point of the eye and are approaching the inner corner, turn the pencil so that you are drawing from underneath on the inner rim, so that the line tapers off at the right point.

» For the lower lash line, draw right on the edge of the rim – not on it, since that makes eyes look smaller.

» The golden rule for good make-up is never to have a hard line. Use a smudger or your little finger to soften the line.

TIPS AND HINTS FOR EYELINER

» Experiment with colours other than brown and black – eyeliner can complement or contrast with your eyeshadow. Grey can be very effective, while green, purple and blue freshen a look.

» Eyeliner worked in between the roots of the lashes will make them look thicker.

» Nude eyeliner pencil around the inner rim of the eyes makes eyes appear rounder. Dark colour on the inner rim elongates the eyes, making them seem narrower. This gives a sultry look, but it will make eyes appear smaller. Don't use any eyeliner other than pencil on the inner rim of your eyes.

» If you have close-set eyes, keeping eyeliner to the outer corners, from the mid point, will be more flattering than if you draw the line all the way to the nose.

eyeshadow

Eyeshadow formulations are so sophisticated that whatever texture and finish you choose, you can be confident that the colour will glide on effortlessly and adhere to the lid without creasing or flaking. Jet-milled powders and pigments mean that metallic and shimmery shadows can be worn without risk of them settling into fine lines. Creamy eye crayons offer a foolproof way to experiment with colour and are convenient to use on the go. Crème and silk shadows containing moisturizing antiageing properties provide the benefits of skincare while giving a sheer wash of colour.

POWDER SHADOWS Available in endless colours and finishes from matte to metallic, powder shadows are long-lasting and versatile, allowing you to create many different looks. Apply with a natural brush for the best result.
1 Use a highlight colour over the whole eye area, blending it up to the browbone and out to the outer corner.
2 Either: Apply a mid colour at the lash line and blend it up to the socket crease but not beyond – don't apply the colour at the socket, or you will have to blend it too far beyond. For a deeper intensity of colour, apply another layer of colour at the lash line and blend it up to the socket, making the colour more intense at the outer corner of the eye if you wish.
Or: Define the socket to add extra drama. Using a socket brush, apply a deep or mid colour to the centre of the hollow of the socket, right in the middle of the crease, and blend it horizontally in both directions using small circular motions, fading the colour towards the inner and outer corners of the eye. Be careful not to go too far – the colour should not come right down to the inner or outer corners of the eye. You should see a soft halo of colour when your eye is open.
3 Sweep an extra layer of highlighter under the browbone.

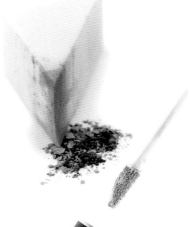
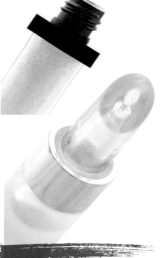

'Whether you're going for dramatic statement or subtle enhancement, the secret for successful eyeshadow application is to blend, blend, blend.'

CRÈME SHADOWS These give a subtle, natural finish and work well with dewy foundation. Crème shadow tends not to be as long-lasting as powder or crayon, so you will need to touch it up. You can apply it with a synthetic brush or your finger.

SILK AND GEL SHADOWS Silk and gel give a wash of colour with a dewy finish. They often come with a wand applicator and can be blended with your finger.

EYE CRAYONS These come in many colours, in metallic, shimmery or matte finishes.
1 Draw along the upper lash line, working colour between the roots of the lashes as if it were an oversized eyeliner, then colour in the lid up to the socket crease.
2 Using your finger or a brush, soften and smudge the edge so that colour blurs a tiny way beyond the socket crease.
3 Draw with light feathery motions on the lower lash line, working the colour under the root of the lashes. Soften the lower edge of the line with your finger.
4 Lightly dust with translucent powder to set.

TIPS AND HINTS FOR EYESHADOW

Make sure brows are well tweezed, as any hairs on the eyelid will trap eyeshadow and make blending difficult.

Dab a little foundation or concealer over the eyelids to hide any redness and create a smooth base. If you are using a crème, silk or crayon eyeshadow, apply it on top. If you are using powder eyeshadow, brush the eyelid with a little translucent powder to absorb moisture first.

Use a lighter shade over the whole eye before applying a darker colour. Always apply at the point where you want the darkest colour, whether that's at the root of the lashes or the crease of the socket line, and then blend. Apply a little highlight colour along the browbone.

Light-reflecting or pearlized shadows swept up to the browbone and dotted in the inner corner of the eye will open up the eyes and make them look brighter.

Shimmery textures give your eyes a twinkly glow; in natural shades, they make tired eyes look more awake.

Don't be afraid to mix textures and finishes – matte and frost can be used together, glitter and some shimmery powders can be blended over crèmes, and a layer of gloss can be applied over powder shadow.

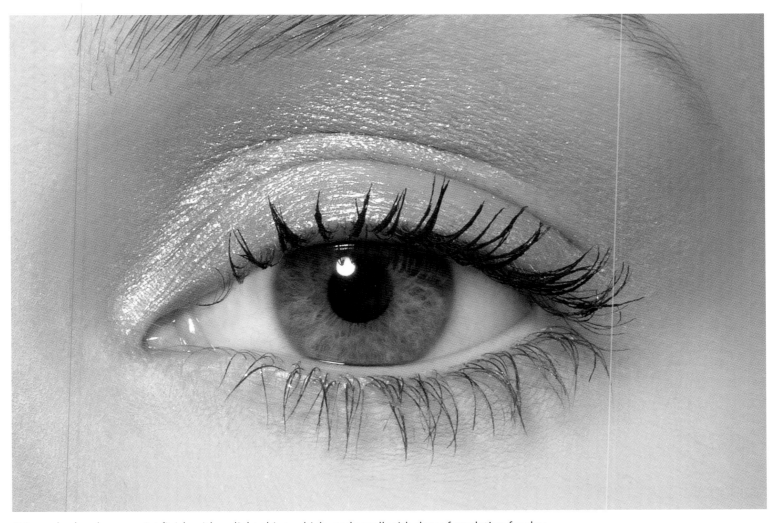

Crème shadow has a moist finish with a slight shine, which works well with dewy foundation for day.

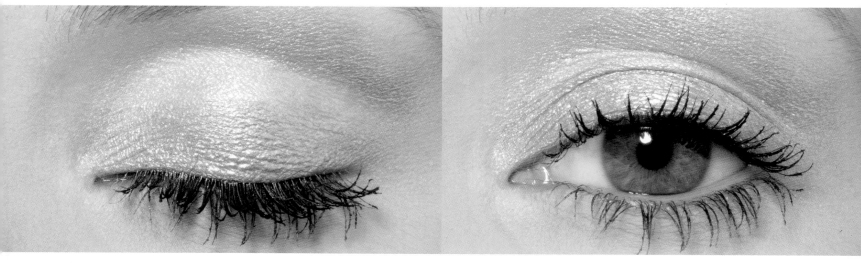

Sheer shadow gives a delicate wash of colour all over the eye. Apply it from the lash line to the browbone.

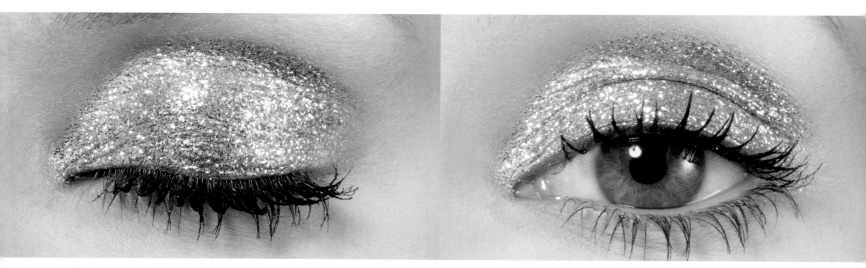

Glitter creates a dramatic sparkle for a fun night-time look. It needs to be applied on top of crème shadow so that it has something to adhere to.

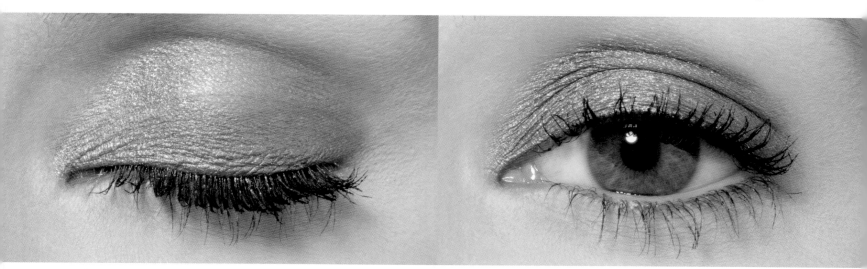

Loose metallic pigment gives an intensity of colour that is great for evening glamour.

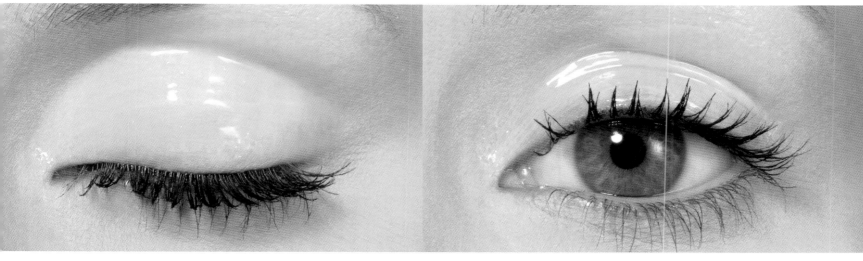

Gloss can be used on its own or over coloured powder shadow for a shiny finish. It can feel sticky and works best on a big lid that isn't hooded.

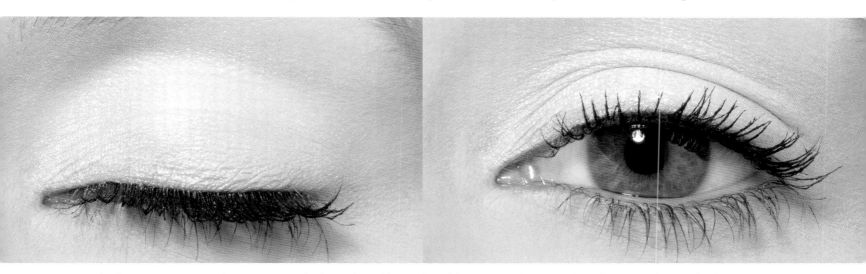

Frost eyeshadow creates a great day-to-evening look. Apply it all over the lid from the lash line and blend it out and up to the browbone.

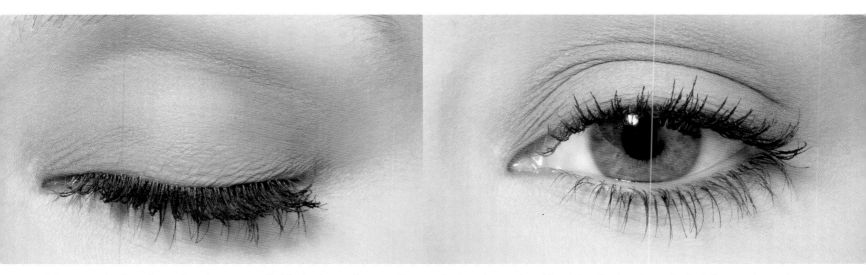

Matte eyeshadow gives a heavier, opaque finish. Apply a pale neutral up to the browbone, then blend the shadow from the lash line to the socket.

step-by-step guide to perfect eyeshadow

Whatever palette you choose, here's a guide to applying eyeshadow using three toning shades – highlight, mid and defining colour. This method applies whether you're using neutral cream, taupe and brown for a natural daytime look or a more dramatic combination of pale lilac, plum and amethyst for night-time glamour.

Choose good-quality brushes for dense application of colour and smooth blending. Use a small brush for applying the colour and a slightly larger, wider brush for blending it. Natural hair is best for applying powder shadow; a good brush with densely packed bristles can be washed frequently without shedding.

'Add colour gradually, building up intensity as required. Always apply dark colour below the point where you want it to end, and blend up and out.'

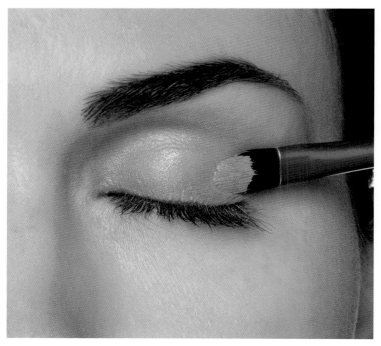

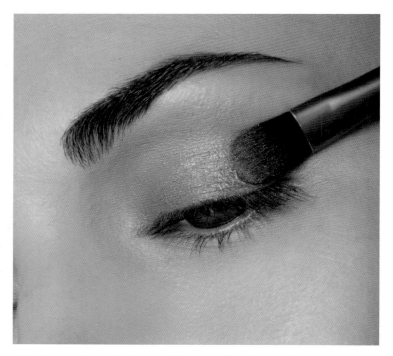

1 Prep the eyes and create a neutral base. Using a firm synthetic brush or your fingertip, dot a little foundation or concealer over the eyelid and blend to the browbone. This will camouflage any blue or red undertones and create a smooth surface. If you're using powder eyeshadow, lightly dust the eyelid with translucent powder to absorb any surface oils and ensure smooth blending.

2 Load a medium-sized natural-hair eye brush with the mid colour and tap off any excess. Starting at the outer corner of the eyelid, blend the shadow all over the eyelid from the lash line to the socket, creating a semicircle of colour.

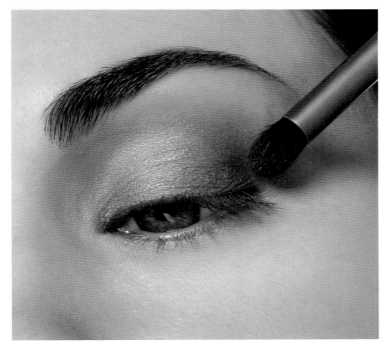

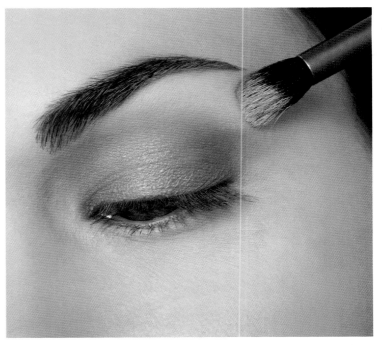

3 Use a smaller, rounder brush to add a little of the deeper defining colour in the hollow of the socket, blending it out to the outer corner of the eye and blurring the edges for a soft, smouldering effect. Build up colour gradually to the desired intensity.

4 Use a small blending brush to sweep highlighter over the arch of the browbone.

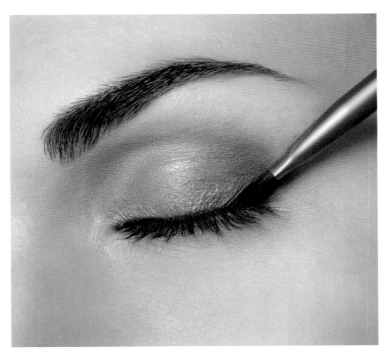

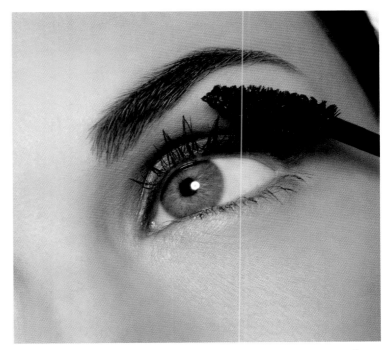

5 Using a small pointed brush, define the upper lash line with the darker shadow, working the colour between the roots of the lashes. (You can achieve a similar effect using an eyeliner pencil and softly blurring the line with a smudger.)

6 Define the upper and lower lashes with mascara (see page 100).

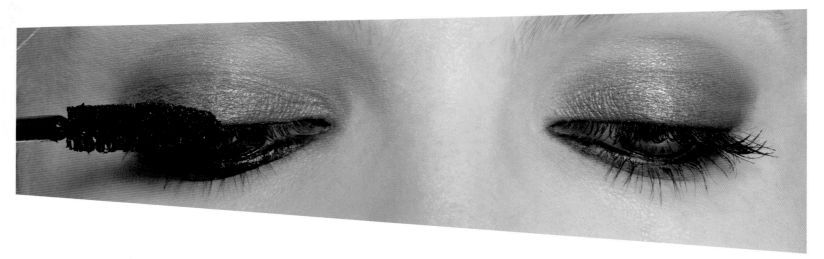

step-by-step guide to smoky eyes

Sultry and super-sexy, smoky eyes is one of the most popular evening looks and the one I am most often asked how to do. Depending on your mood, you can tone it down for a more wearable, sophisticated version, or max out the kohl to make it more edgy and rock-chick. Don't feel limited to a palette of charcoal and grey – chocolate browns, deep berry colours, midnight blues and metallic gunmetal and silver can all work extremely well.

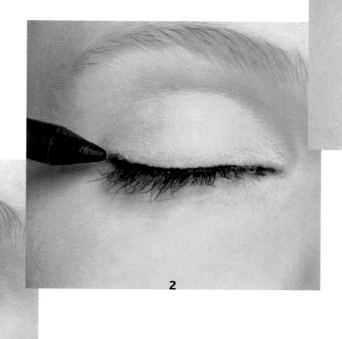

1

2

3

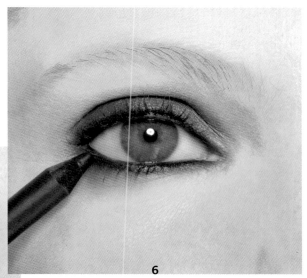

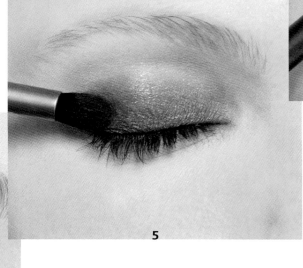

1 Prep the eyelids with a neutral base of foundation or concealer set with a light dusting of translucent powder. Starting at the outer corner of the upper lash line, push the tip of a black eyeliner pencil between the roots of the lashes.

2 Work all the way along the upper lash line, building up colour intensity between and around the lashes. This gives depth of colour and makes the lashes look thicker.

3 Using a small, pointed natural-hair brush, blend dark grey eyeshadow along the upper lash line, smudging the pencil and blending it all together.

4 Using a synthetic brush, apply silvery grey crème eyeshadow above the eyeliner, blending it up to the socket crease. This creates a creamy base for the powder eyeshadow to adhere to and intensifies the effect.

5 Using a natural-hair brush, blend a little more dark grey powder eyeshadow over the lower part of the lid, blending it from the lash line upwards and outwards and blurring the colours together.

6 Apply black eyeliner pencil all the way around the inside of the upper lid and along the edge of the lower lid at the roots of the lashes. Finish with lashings of mascara to define the eyes (see opposite, top).

luscious lashes

No eyes are complete without a frame of perfectly curled and defined lashes to flutter. For a semi-permanent solution – ideal for holidays – consider having your lashes permed and dyed, but for every day there are mascaras to colour, thicken, volumize, lengthen, curl or condition. Waterproof formulations withstand rain, tears and swimming – they can be a godsend for wearers of contact lenses. Clear mascara gives a dewy look to natural lashes and can also be used to hold brows in shape.

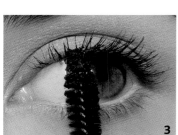

Colour

Black mascara defines the eyes like nothing else and works with almost any look, but electric blues and deep purples can also be stunning, so don't be afraid to experiment. Dark brown mascara is generally softer and more flattering for mature faces.

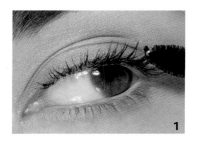

Application

Whatever formulation you choose, here is a foolproof guide to applying mascara:

1 Make sure the wand is not overloaded so that the product is less likely to come into contact with the skin. Look down and stroke the wand over the top of the upper lashes from roots to tips. Move along from one corner of the eye to the other until every lash is coated.

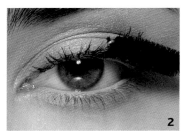

2 With the eyes wide open, stroke the wand up the upper lashes from underneath, starting at the roots and sweeping up to the tips. Move along as before from one corner to the other until every lash is coated. Repeat, but this time move the wand up the lashes in a zigzag motion to coat the sides of each lash.

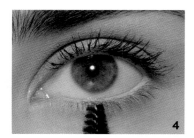

3 To add more volume to the roots of the upper lashes, hold the wand vertically and push it directly up into the roots, working your way along from corner to corner.

4 To coat the lower lashes, hold the wand vertically and sweep it from side to side over the lashes, being careful not to let the wand touch your face.

TOP TIPS

» Remove any unwanted clumps of mascara with an eyelash comb.

» Gently wipe away smudges with a cotton bud dipped in eye make-up remover.

» Don't pump the wand – this traps air and makes the product dry out faster.

» The wand can harbour bacteria, so don't share mascara and discard it after three months – or immediately if you have an eye infection.

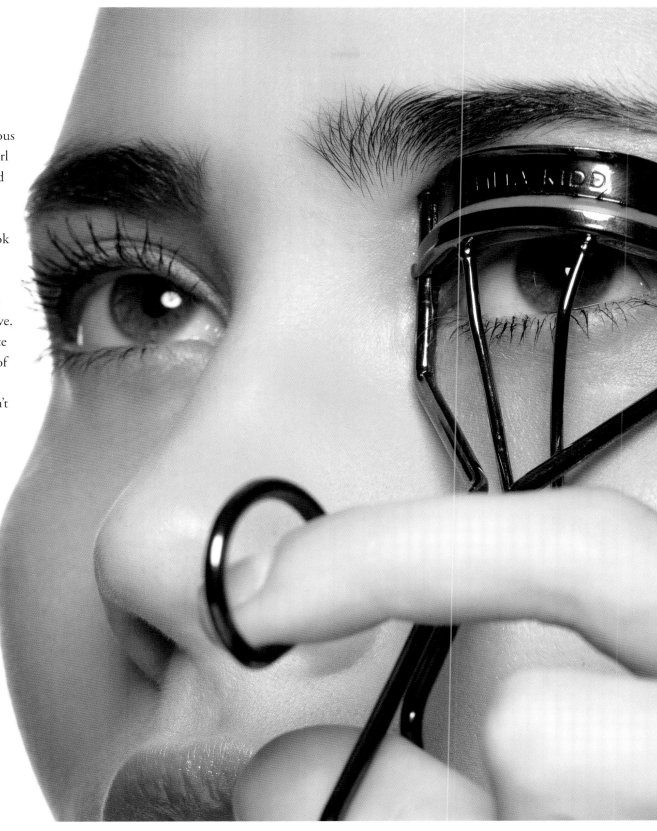

Curl

My top tip for a gorgeous wide-eyed look is to curl your lashes – it lifts and fans them out, really opening up the eyes. Eyelash curlers may look like an instrument of torture, but once you master the art, they are very simple and effective.

1 Look down, and place the curler at the roots of your upper lashes.

2 Making sure you don't catch the eyelid as you clamp down, gently squeeze the curlers onto the lashes close to the roots.

3 Work gradually outwards along the length of the lashes towards the tips, keeping the pressure the same to create an even, gentle curve.

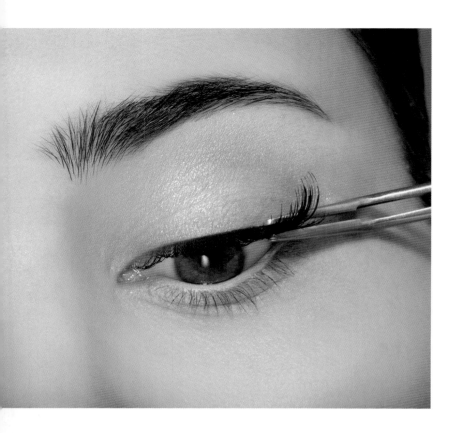

TO APPLY INDIVIDUAL LASHES Put glue on the back of your hand and draw the lash through it. Apply using fingers, tweezers or a false-lash applicator. Use most of the lashes on the outer corner of the eye, working in to about two-thirds of the way along.

TO APPLY A FULL SET Trim the false lashes to the right size for your eye – if they stick out too far at either corner, they are more likely to lift off. If you have short lashes, trim the false ones so that they don't dominate your face. Apply glue at the base – I often use a toothpick or matchstick to make sure the glue is finely but thoroughly applied along the whole length. Press the strip onto your eyelid so that it lies at the roots where your natural lashes grow, with no lid showing in between.

Fake it

False eyelashes create instant glamour for night-time and parties. For a natural look, go for individual or grouped lashes; for faster application, use a full set or a half set on the outer corners of the eyes. Tread carefully if you have a heavy top lid – corner lashes will be more flattering than a full set.

Apply falsies before mascara but after the rest of your eye make-up. Line the eye with liquid eyeliner or a dark pencil to help disguise the glue. Curl your own lashes and use a lash tint or a non-volumizing mascara, which will darken but not thicken them. Don't wait for it to dry – the slight wetness will help the natural and false lashes to lie together evenly.

My secret Rather than trying to get the angle right

TO APPLY HALF LASHES Applied at the outer corner, these create a cat's-eye shape. They should be very fine or the difference between natural and false lashes will be too extreme. Apply as for full lashes, making sure you've trimmed any extra length before you apply the glue.

GENTLY CURL the natural and false lashes together and reapply mascara – just stroking the tips is enough. Thick mascara adds too much volume.

TO REMOVE Support your natural lashes by squeezing both sets together with finger and thumb. With the other hand, gently lift away the base of the false lashes, then carefully pull them away. Cleanse the lashes using an oil-based make-up remover.

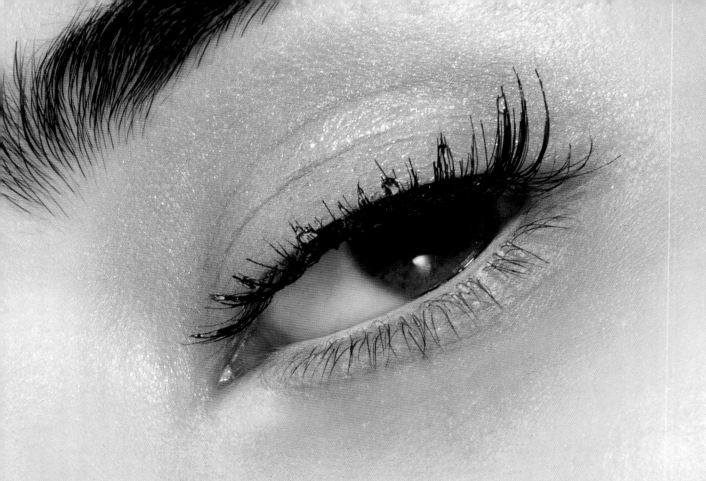

by gluing only the base, I add glue further along the false lashes and press them onto the natural lash to get them lying flat.

TOP TEN EYE LOOKS

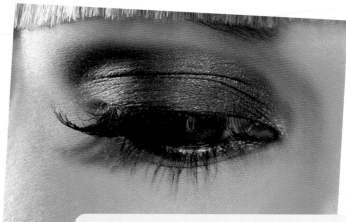

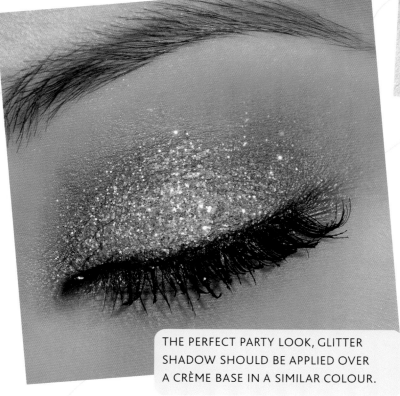

DARK EYES FRINGED WITH HEAVY FALSE LASHES COATED IN THICK MASCARA WAS THE SIGNATURE LOOK OF 1960S MODEL TWIGGY. HERE BLUE METALLIC CRÈME HAS BEEN APPLIED TO THE WHOLE LID AND BLENDED OUTWARDS.

THE PERFECT PARTY LOOK, GLITTER SHADOW SHOULD BE APPLIED OVER A CRÈME BASE IN A SIMILAR COLOUR.

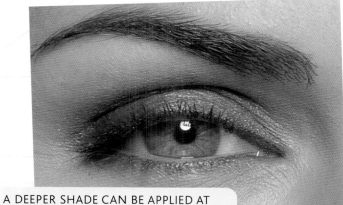

A DEEPER SHADE CAN BE APPLIED AT THE OUTER CORNER OF THE EYE IN THE CREASE OF THE SOCKET FOR ADDED DEPTH AND INTENSITY OF COLOUR.

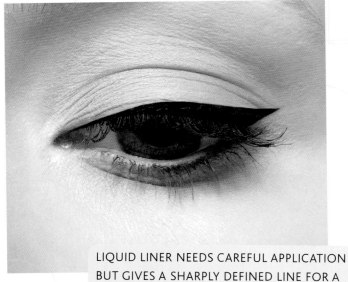

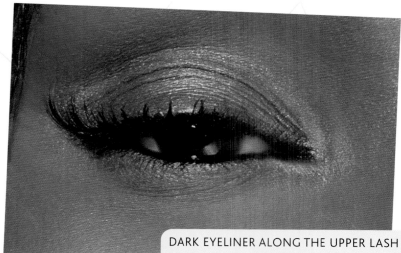

LIQUID LINER NEEDS CAREFUL APPLICATION BUT GIVES A SHARPLY DEFINED LINE FOR A GLAMOROUS FLICK. THE REST OF THE EYE IS NEUTRAL, WITH WHITE EYELINER ALONG THE INNER RIM OF THE LOWER LASH LINE FOR A BRIGHTENING EFFECT.

DARK EYELINER ALONG THE UPPER LASH LINE AND ALONG THE INNER RIM OF THE EYE, EXTENDING AT THE OUTER CORNER, CREATES AN ELONGATED FOCUS, FURTHER ACCENTUATED BY FALSE-LASH CORNERS.

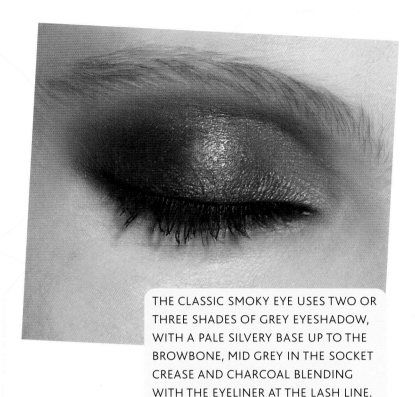

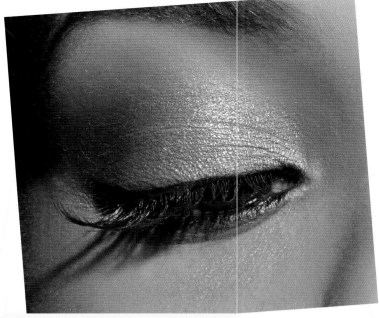

THE CLASSIC SMOKY EYE USES TWO OR THREE SHADES OF GREY EYESHADOW, WITH A PALE SILVERY BASE UP TO THE BROWBONE, MID GREY IN THE SOCKET CREASE AND CHARCOAL BLENDING WITH THE EYELINER AT THE LASH LINE.

FALSE-LASH CORNERS AND THICK BLACK EYELINER ALONG THE UPPER LASH LINE, EXTENDING UPWARDS AT THE OUTER CORNER, CREATE A SEXY CAT'S EYE.

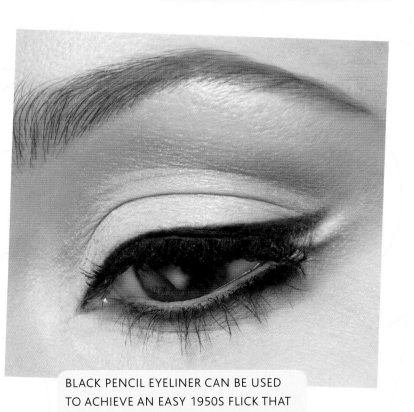

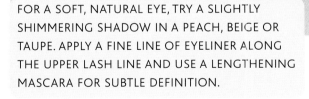

FOR A SOFT, NATURAL EYE, TRY A SLIGHTLY SHIMMERING SHADOW IN A PEACH, BEIGE OR TAUPE. APPLY A FINE LINE OF EYELINER ALONG THE UPPER LASH LINE AND USE A LENGTHENING MASCARA FOR SUBTLE DEFINITION.

BLACK PENCIL EYELINER CAN BE USED TO ACHIEVE AN EASY 1950S FLICK THAT EXTENDS AT THE OUTER CORNERS OF THE EYES WITH SOFTLY SMUDGED EDGES.

SOPHISTICATED BROWN EYESHADOW IS A PERENNIALLY POPULAR DARK NEUTRAL, AS IT WORKS WELL AT ANY AGE AND WITH ANY SKIN TONE AND EYE COLOUR.

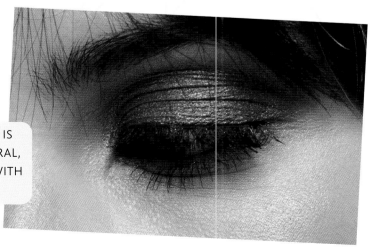

FLAWLESS FACE

With the right products and techniques, it isn't hard to achieve a flawless, radiant complexion, and today's high-tech foundations, concealers and powders produce astonishingly natural results.

What coverage do I need?

GOOD CLEAR SKIN Liquid sheer foundation or tinted moisturizer provide the lightest, barely-there coverage that evens out skin tone and gives extra radiance.

THE ODD TROUBLE SPOT Heavier liquid foundations or crème-to-powder formulations offer slightly more coverage.

PROBLEM SKIN Crème or stick foundations give full natural coverage and are suitable for hyperpigmented or scarred skin.

Foundation is your canvas, so invest in a good formulation that's right for your skin. Today's foundations are multipurpose, offering far more than colour correction and coverage, with built-in sun protection, moisturizers and antiageing ingredients. They allow skin to breathe, while protecting it from the elements and environmental pollutants. Formulations containing silicones glide on without giving a mask-like look and enhance the quality of the skin. Light-reflecting particles bounce light away from surface lines to create a radiant airbrushed glow.

Textures

Check the ingredients and select the correct formulation for your skin with added vitamins and moisturizers. Choose talc-free foundation that soaks in easily – nothing with a thick, powdery finish. A moisturizing foundation is essential for dry skin, whereas an oil-free, matte finish is ideal for oily skin. Mature women need a little shimmer in their foundation to bring light to their skin, but anyone with scarring or acne should avoid light-reflecting particles as they can emphasize blemishes. A light-coverage liquid foundation is best for normal skin and tinted moisturizer is a good choice for summer.

Colour-matching foundation

The right shade of foundation should disappear into your skin seamlessly. Match the colour around your nose and sweep across the apple of your cheek.

» Check the colour in natural light – artificial light is deceptive and what looks right at the make-up counter can look very unnatural in daylight.

» Never use foundation to change your skin tone – foundation should have the same colour base as your skin (see pages 36–7).

» Don't forget that your skin is a different colour in summer and winter and you should change your shade of foundation accordingly. If you buy two shades, you can mix them together for a perfect match all year round.

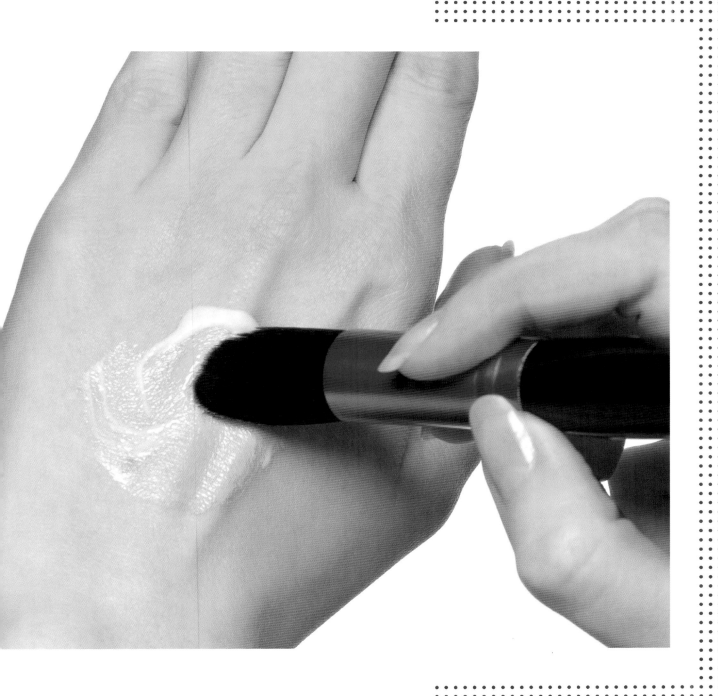

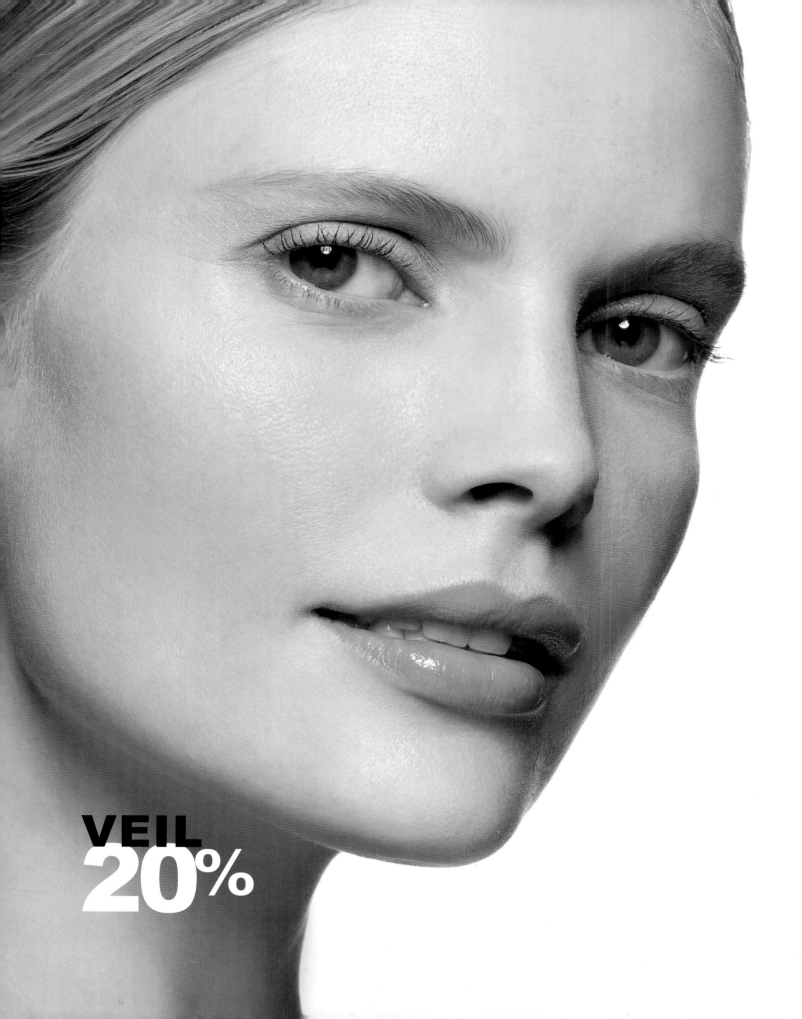

VEIL
20%

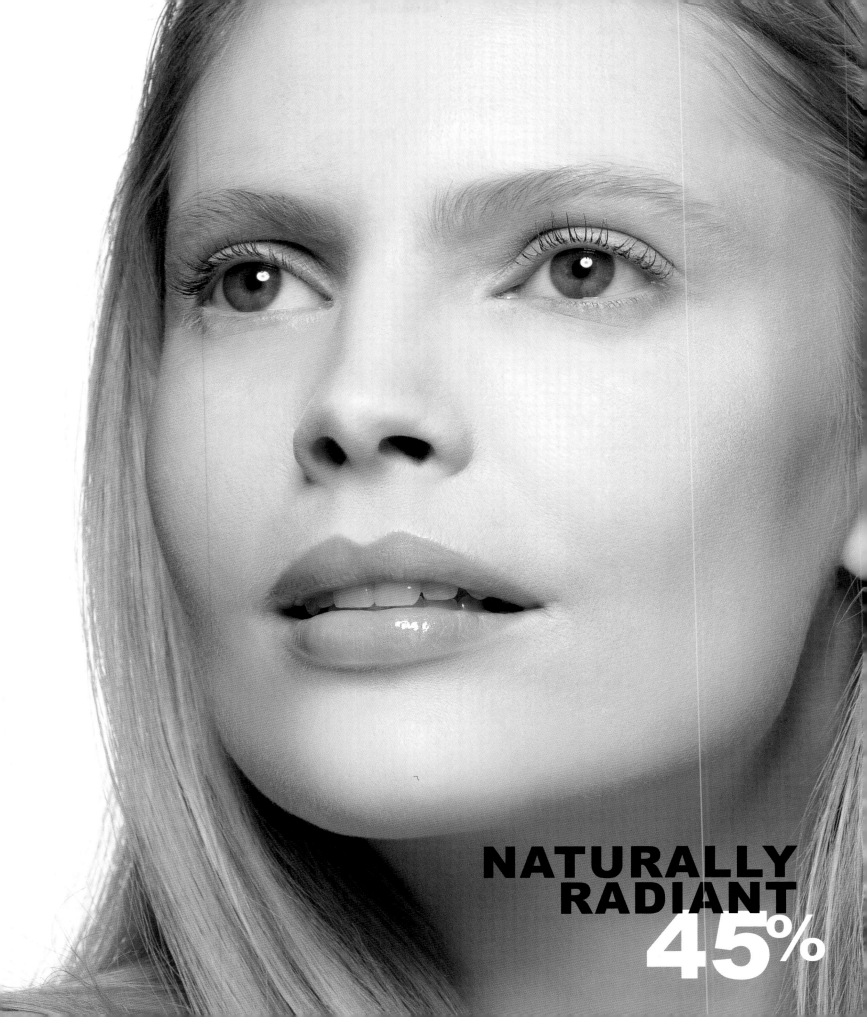

NATURALLY RADIANT
45%

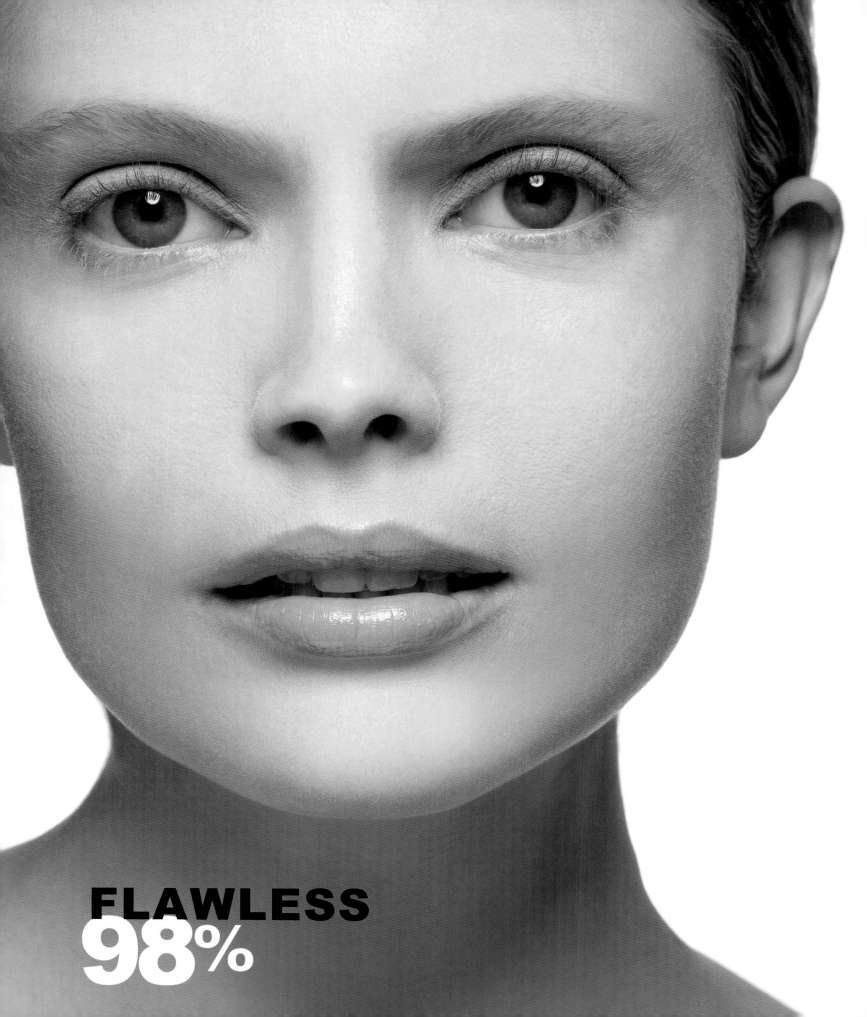

FLAWLESS
98%

Veil

This is the lightest form of almost transparent coverage, which allows the skin to show through and simply evens out tone and gives an extra glow. This sheer finish is achieved with tinted moisturizer, which is ideal for young healthy complexions and is also a good option in the summer when a light, dewy base is often desired. Tinted moisturizer usually comes in only three or four shades – from light through medium to dark. Choose the shade that's closest to your skin tone, but because the formulation is so light and sheer it's hard to go wrong – you can get away with one that is as much as two shades darker. Smooth tinted moisturizer all over the face, pressing it into the skin rather than wiping it on and off. Use a very light wax-based concealer to disguise any areas of redness or dark shadows under the eyes.

Naturally radiant

To create a luminous natural semi-matte complexion that is perfect for every day, use a light hydrating foundation containing light-reflecting particles. Apply the foundation only where you need it to even out the skin tone – around the nose, on the nose bridge, cheekbones and chin. Use a pointed synthetic brush to press the product into the skin and blend it well. Use concealer to build up extra opacity where you need it. For evening or a more luminous dewy glow, blend crème highlighter along the cheekbones, browbone and collarbone. Then set with the lightest dusting of very fine talc-free translucent powder. If your skin is oily, mineral make-up applied with a flat-topped natural-hair polishing brush would achieve a similar naturally radiant base.

Flawless

Unless you have problem skin, this maximum-perfection coverage is best reserved for night-time when you want a really flawless finish – think full-scale screen-siren glamour. Matte foundation is applied all over the skin with a pointed synthetic brush. Perfectly colour-matched concealer is then used to colour-correct under the eyes and around the sides of the nostrils, and to hide any blemishes and flaws, with special care taken to ensure it is fully worked in so as to avoid creasing. To finish, the make-up is set with very fine talc-free translucent powder.

FOUNDATION APPLICATION

Always prepare your skin properly before you start. Foundation applied to dry skin quickly looks flaky. Powder on top makes it worse and blending blush becomes impossible.

Apply an appropriate moisturizer for your skin and let it sink in for five minutes before applying foundation – this will prevent a patchy finish. This is especially relevant if you are using a crème foundation, which tends to cake if skin is even slightly dry.

Using a primer will help make-up to last longer and is particularly good if you have skin that absorbs make-up. It helps to even out skin tone and provides a perfect base for foundation. Don't use a primer as a substitute for moisturizer, though.

Apply foundation only on the areas that need it to even out skin tone – around the nose, chin or cheeks. Use a dabbing motion that pushes the product into the skin rather than wiping it on and off in the same movement – a foundation brush, sponge or fingers are all fine.

As with all make-up, blend, blend, blend, making sure you work foundation into any creases and being careful to avoid tidemarks at the jaw and hairline.

concealer

The golden rule for concealer is to choose the right shade for your skin tone and the correct texture for whatever you're attempting to disguise. Get either of these wrong and your concealer will only draw attention to the blemish.

Concealers come in many tones and textures, from liquids and creams to sticks and compacts. I favour a creamy texture that adheres well to the skin, so reducing the risk of it rubbing off. A moisturizing formulation sinks in and won't dry to a powdery finish; it's also easy to apply and blend.

The best concealers, available in shades for light to dark skin tones, come in a compact of two colours that can be used individually, layered to build up cover or blended for a perfect colour-match. Use the lighter, pinker colour to cover dark undereye circles, which have a blue undertone, and the yellow-toned flesh colour to conceal spots and broken capillaries, which have red undertones.

Colour-matching concealer

» Colour-match in natural light. Blend a little concealer around your nostril: the correct shade will disappear into your skin.

» Make sure the concealer is not too light for your skin, as this will accentuate blemishes and dark circles.

» Liquid concealers are the sheerest and are ideal if you have very fair skin.

» If your skin is medium to dark, creamier compact or stick concealers will tend to work better.

CONCEALER APPLICATION

Using a stiff flat synthetic brush or the pad of your finger, press concealer into the skin with firm pats. Use a twisting motion to work it into the skin and ensure you are not wiping it on and then off.

For very light coverage, use concealer on its own without foundation. Cover a spot or any patches of discoloration with concealer, then set with a light dusting of sheer translucent powder.

For more coverage, apply foundation and let it soak into the skin. Then apply the concealer, patting it in very lightly to avoid wiping off the foundation underneath. Blend the edges well and set with powder.

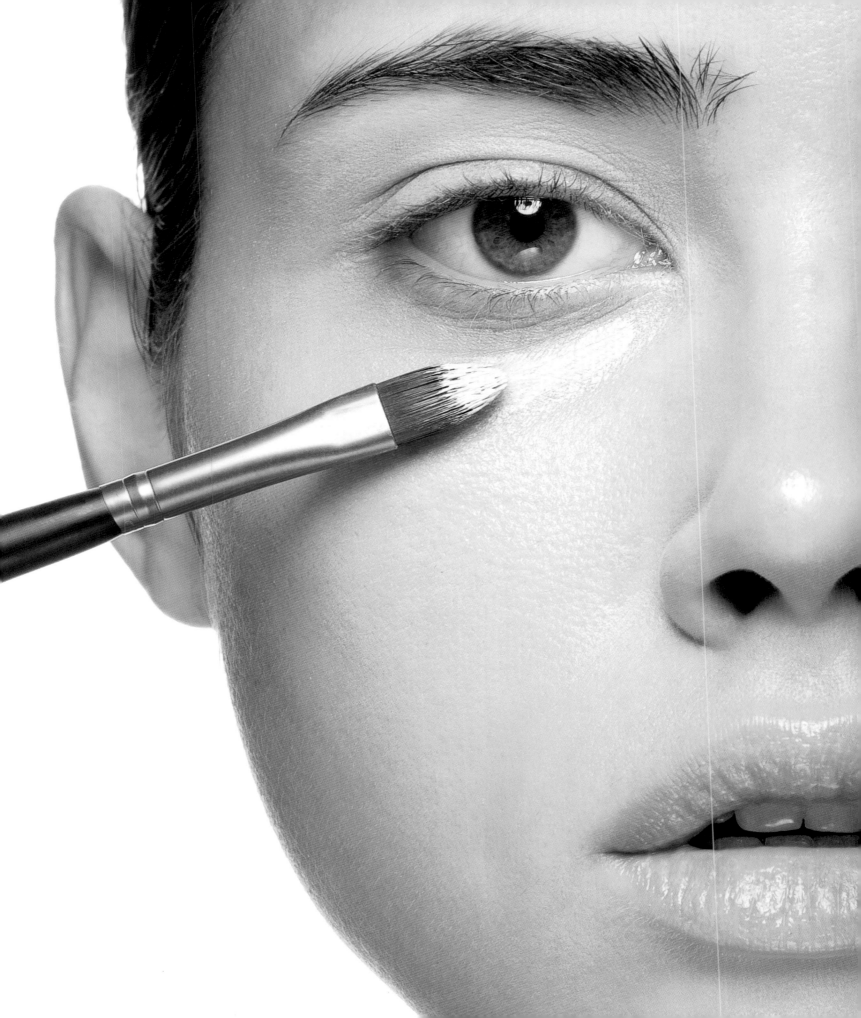

Spots

There are hundreds of products aimed at healing spots, but none makes them disappear instantly. That's where make-up comes in, but take care – a badly covered spot is more noticeable than one left bare.

» No squeezing! Squeezing blackheads will enlarge the pores, while spots become inflamed and take longer to heal. For blackheads use clay or hot masks to draw out impurities, and for others invest in good cleansers and antibacterial wands.

» Use a firm creamy concealer – anything that dries to a powdery finish will look flaky and make the spot obvious. If you have a raised pimple, use a yellow-toned concealer that's slightly darker than your skin.

» Dab the concealer on with your finger or a brush. Once the spot is covered, don't touch, or you'll wipe the concealer off the top. Blend the edges around the pimple into the skin.

» Gently apply foundation, covering the blended edges of the concealer. Leave to absorb and then set with ultra-fine powder – a slightly darker powder than you normally wear can work well to set the concealer.

» To retouch, make sure you have clean hands, then dab concealer on the pimple and blend the edges. Reset with powder, then leave well alone.

Dark circles

The telltale signs of late nights or overindulging, dark undereye circles take away our sparkle. Here's what to do:

» Wrap a little grated raw potato in a muslin cloth, or slice a kiwi. Lie down, and apply to the eye area for 15 minutes. Pat dry.

» Apply a light eye cream containing vitamin K (used by cosmetic surgeons because it prevents bruising), peptides or kinetin.

» Depending on your skin tone, try a concealer with a pink, peach or yellow undertone to neutralize the blue and green in the undereye circles. Light-reflecting ingredients will help to downplay dark circles.

» Avoid plum, purple and red eyeshadows, or you'll look as if you've got black eyes.

Eye bags

Puffy eyes are an indicator of fluid retention and a build-up of toxins in the undereye tissue caused by slow lymphatic drainage. Here's what to do:

» In the long term, cut down on caffeine, alcohol and salt, eat more fresh fruit and veg, and drink plenty of water.

» Use an eye cream formulated to promote fluid drainage. A cold teabag, slice of cucumber or crushed ice wrapped in a muslin cloth can also help to reduce puffiness.

» After overindulging, sleep with an extra pillow – the additional height will help to promote lymphatic drainage and prevent fluid from accumulating.

» Avoid rich eye creams, which could cause congestion, or any that contain ingredients that might irritate.

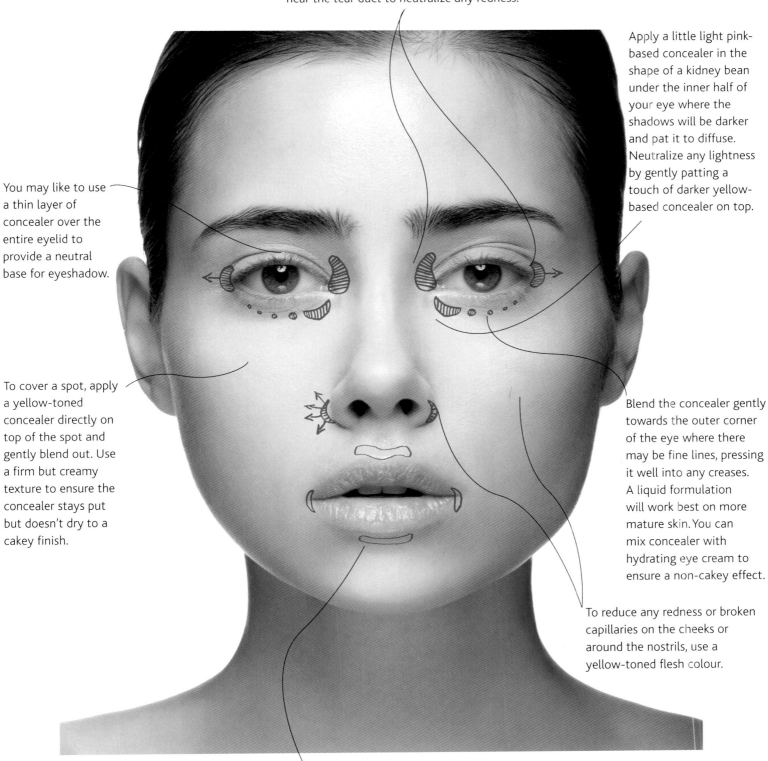

Add a touch of concealer to the outer corner of the eyelids and to the inner corner of the eye near the tear duct to neutralize any redness.

Apply a little light pink-based concealer in the shape of a kidney bean under the inner half of your eye where the shadows will be darker and pat it to diffuse. Neutralize any lightness by gently patting a touch of darker yellow-based concealer on top.

You may like to use a thin layer of concealer over the entire eyelid to provide a neutral base for eyeshadow.

To cover a spot, apply a yellow-toned concealer directly on top of the spot and gently blend out. Use a firm but creamy texture to ensure the concealer stays put but doesn't dry to a cakey finish.

Blend the concealer gently towards the outer corner of the eye where there may be fine lines, pressing it well into any creases. A liquid formulation will work best on more mature skin. You can mix concealer with hydrating eye cream to ensure a non-cakey effect.

To reduce any redness or broken capillaries on the cheeks or around the nostrils, use a yellow-toned flesh colour.

Apply a little concealer around the corners of the lips, under the bottom lip and at the top of the Cupid's bow.

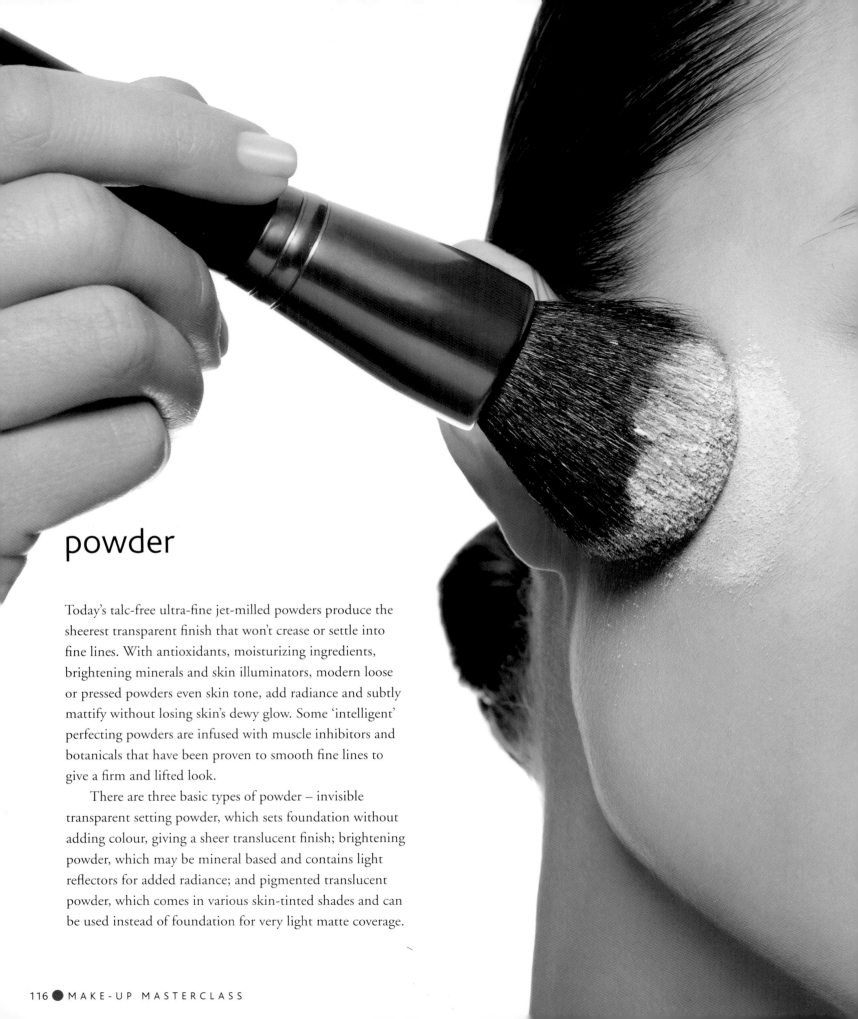

powder

Today's talc-free ultra-fine jet-milled powders produce the sheerest transparent finish that won't crease or settle into fine lines. With antioxidants, moisturizing ingredients, brightening minerals and skin illuminators, modern loose or pressed powders even skin tone, add radiance and subtly mattify without losing skin's dewy glow. Some 'intelligent' perfecting powders are infused with muscle inhibitors and botanicals that have been proven to smooth fine lines to give a firm and lifted look.

There are three basic types of powder – invisible transparent setting powder, which sets foundation without adding colour, giving a sheer translucent finish; brightening powder, which may be mineral based and contains light reflectors for added radiance; and pigmented translucent powder, which comes in various skin-tinted shades and can be used instead of foundation for very light matte coverage.

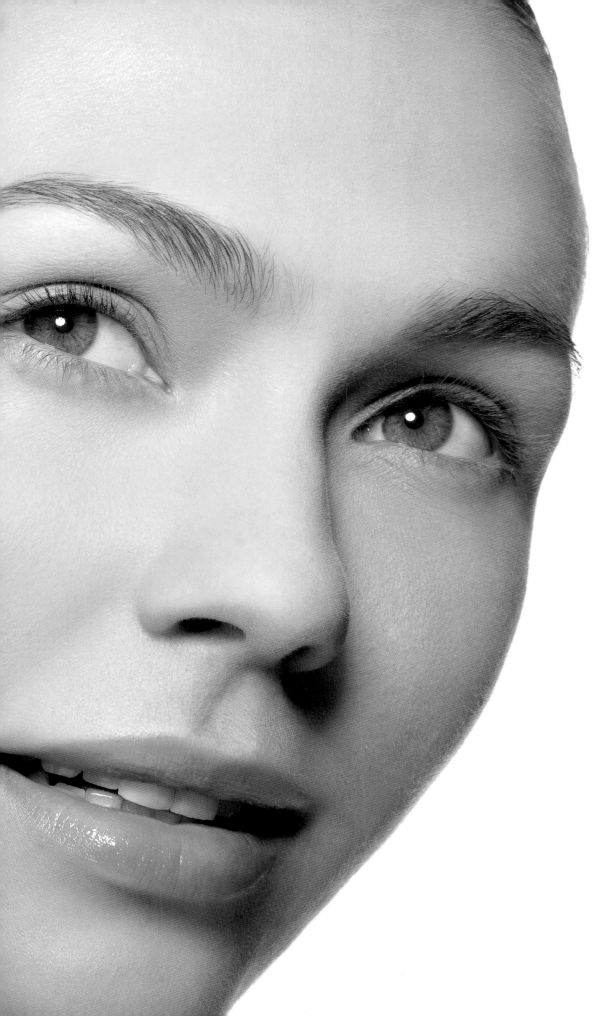

POWDER APPLICATION

» Use a fat brush with soft dense natural bristles. Dip the brush lightly into the powder and blow or tap off the excess. Sweep it lightly over your face to set foundation.

» If you are prone to shine, the area to focus on with a smaller brush is the central cross of the face (see below). Load the brush with powder and tap off the excess, then work it into the skin with a polishing action, using small circular motions.

» Be careful when applying powder under the eyes. Use a small brush and stretch the skin gently with your fingers to ensure the powder is blended and doesn't exaggerate fine lines.

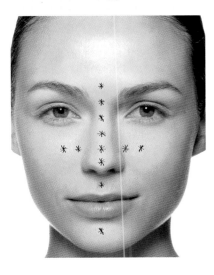

highlighting

Light colours highlight and draw areas forward, while dark colours shade and push them back. Employing these techniques together lets you manipulate light and shadow on your face to create illusions.

Use highlighter on the higher planes of the face, such as cheekbones, browbone, nose, chin, under the eyes, inside the tear ducts and the Cupid's bow of the lips – the idea is to mimic the effect of light on the face. Apply crème highlighter with your finger or a synthetic brush and apply powder with a natural-hair brush.

The tools

Crème and powder highlighters are available for fair skin, but if you have dark skin use a foundation two shades lighter than usual. Highlighters can be matte or shimmery, with light reflectors for extra luminosity, but those with a very high shimmer aren't subtle enough for a lot of contouring work. Instead, mix bone powder eyeshadow with translucent powder to make the required natural tone. Apply crème with a finger, sponge or synthetic brush; use a medium-sized natural-hair cheek brush for powder and a larger brush for blending.

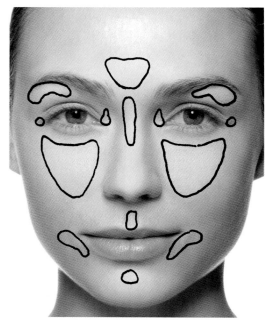

The face map above illustrates the higher planes of the face that would naturally catch the light. Apply highlighter sparingly and blend it well.

My secret A touch of non-shimmery highlighter at the outer corners of the eye and lips will give the face a slight lift.

Cheekbones

Apply highlighter on top of the cheekbone and up the outer edge of the eye socket. Highlighting under the hollow on the back third of the jaw will make the hollow appear deeper and the cheekbone more prominent. Shimmering products are fine to use on the cheekbone itself and the look can be intensified by layering a crème with a high-shimmer powder. Don't take this more intense shimmer up the side of the eyes and use only a pale contouring powder or crème on the jawbone – shimmer will attract too much attention.

Nose

A heavy brow ridge can cast a shadow on the nose bridge, which looks as if you are frowning. Place highlighter on the deepest part of the shadow and soften by blending at each edge. A shimmer product is inappropriate, so look for a light foundation or powder. Don't blend highlighter too high or the correction effect will be lost. A touch of highlighter down the centre of the nose will make a wide nose look narrower, but be careful not to extend it to the rounded tip.

Jawbone

A sagging jawline can be given a crisper edge by applying highlighter at the front of the jaw (behind the chin) and blending out about two-thirds of the way back. Once again, any shimmer will look obvious.

Collarbone

Dab shimmering highlighter along the centre of the collarbone. The effect can be slimming and will draw attention to the décolletage, while also subtly emphasizing cleavage.

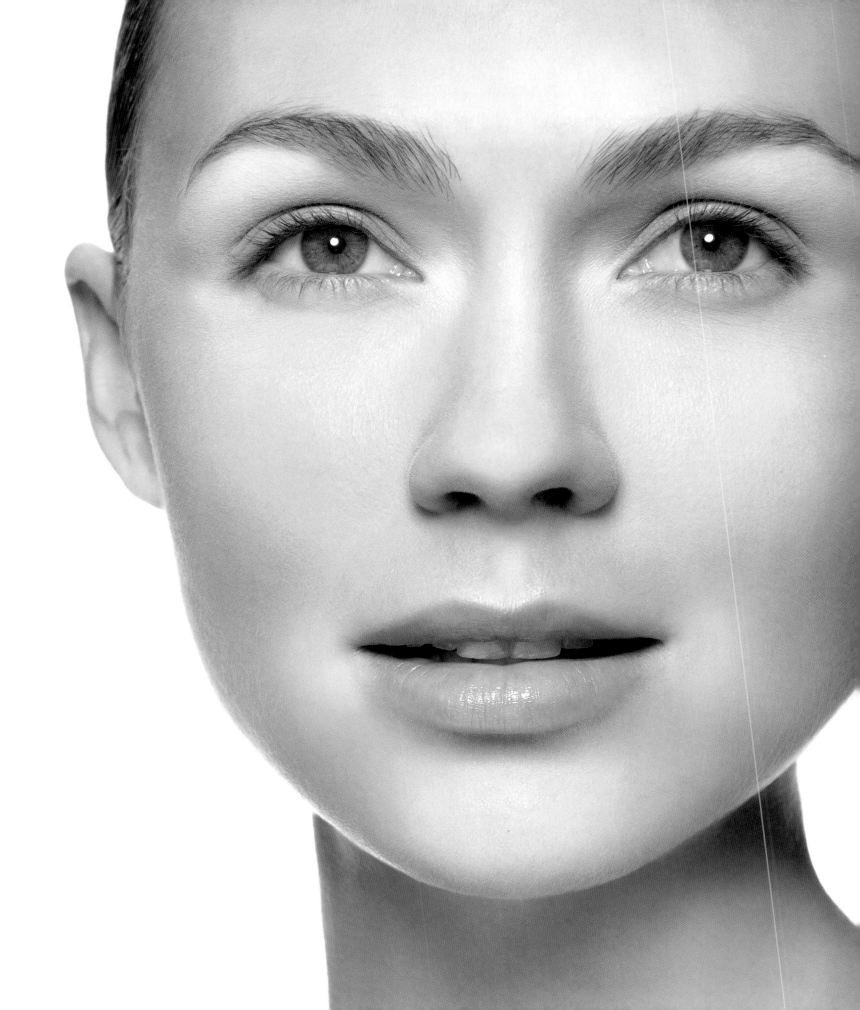

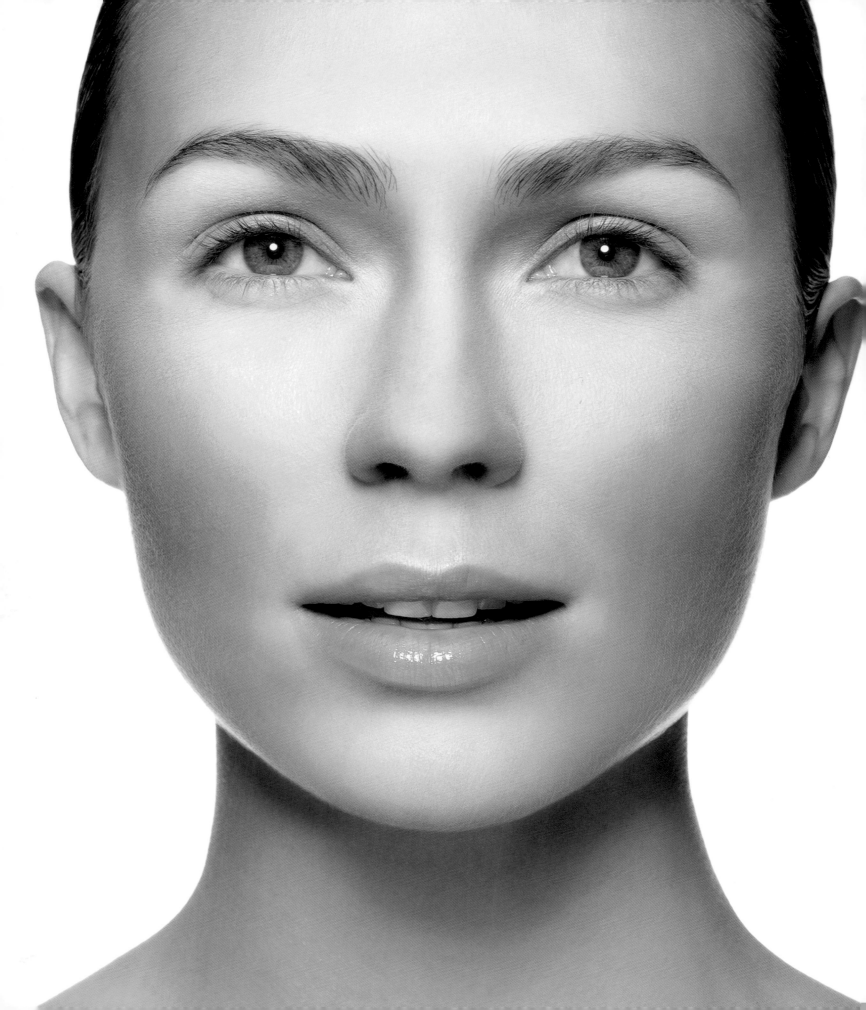

contouring

This technique is often talked about but little understood. Done badly, it can look as if lines have been 'drawn' on the face, but when it is done well, the shape of the face is subtly altered. Remember: the job of make-up is to emphasize individual beauty, not make every face conform to a perfect oval.

The opposite of highlighting, where a lighter colour is used to draw out or bring forward, contouring uses a darker colour to hollow or recede. The two techniques work in combination, but you don't have to highlight right next to a shaded area, since the normal will already seem more prominent by comparison.

The tools

Use foundation or powder two shades darker than your skin tone. If you use a bronzer or powder eyeshadow for this, be careful it doesn't contain too much shimmer – it should have the same luminosity as skin, so it shouldn't be completely matte, either. Apply with an oval-headed cheek brush or a sponge and use a larger brush for blending.

The technique

Be precise in application, then blend. Bones are curved, so shadows are, too – a hard edge looks false, while any shadow that goes beyond the point you want to deepen will destroy the illusion. Start with very little product and add more as required.

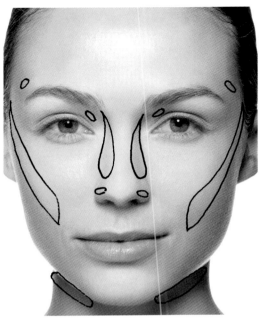

The face map represents the parts of the face that would fall into shadow if light were shone on it. Contouring adds definition to the face and subtly alters its shape.

My secret This technique requires practice. I teach my professional students using black and white. Once they have mastered the theory and techniques, we go on to use natural colours.

Cheekbones

Suck in your cheeks to find your natural hollow. This can be emphasized by shading the area with a tadpole shape – the 'head' in the hollow under the cheek apple, the 'tail' blending to nothing towards the hairline. The contouring should not be too low, just on the underside of the bone.

Balance this with a dot at the hollow of each temple and blend. A wide forehead can be slimmed by shading at the temple hollow towards the hairline.

Nose

To slim a wide nose, shade either side, starting from below the bridge and ending above the nostrils. A flared or bulbous nose needs a touch of shade only at either side of the tip. Those with very flat noses can add a shadow at the inner corner of the eye.

Jawline

Those with a droop, should shade just below the jawline and blend upwards to the edge. A square jaw can be shaded at the corner under the earlobe, blending out to remove an impression of overheaviness. Contouring under the jawbone will define the jawline and slim the neck.

CHARMING CHEEKS

A pretty flush creates youthful radiance and makes you glow with vitality. As well as brightening the complexion with a pop of colour, blush enhances face shape and emphasizes the cheekbones.

The colour you choose – from fresh pink or soft peach to deep plum, tawny brown or bronze – makes all the difference to your finished look. If you have very pale skin, shades such as clear rose and pale apricot give a gentle flush. If you have dark skin, try intense shades such as raspberry pink and coral, or deep bronze and gold. Don't be put off by how the colour looks in the palette – it will often give a very different effect blended on skin.

Some palettes contain two complementary shades – a soft neutral that works well for everyday or for contouring, and a brighter shade that can be used to add freshness or drama. The softer, deeper colour can be swept into the hollow below the cheekbones for subtle shading and a little used at the temples for balance. The fresher, brighter shade can then be applied to the apples of the cheeks and blended up along the cheekbones. You can also layer the two to create the perfect depth of colour for your skin.

As your skin tone deepens through the summer, you should alter the colour and even the texture of your blush. Very sheer crème, gel, mousse or liquid blushes look more natural than powder blush in the summer light. These can be worn on bare, moisturized skin, or over tinted moisturizer or light liquid foundation.

My secret Use a similar colour for your lips but in a darker or lighter shade, not exactly matching.

TOP TIPS

» Choose a blush that adds life to your complexion.

» If you're very fair, stick to light fresh pink, pale peach or tawny tones.

» The darker your colouring, the more blush you need and the more striking the colours you can get away with.

» Peach is a flattering shade all year round and suits a variety of skin tones and ages – the only skin it doesn't suit is tanned or sallow. Even those with red cheeks can wear peach because the yellow undertone helps to correct this.

» You can always mix colours to get the perfect shade and depth.

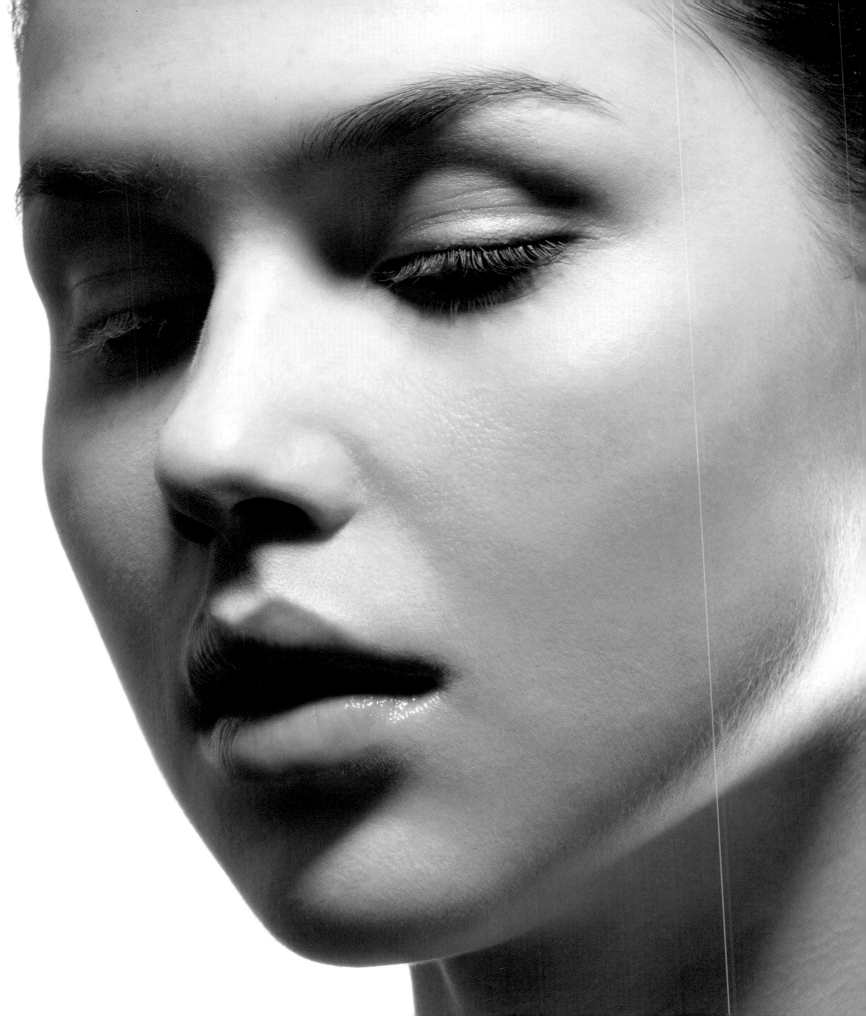

BLUSH APPLICATION

Well-applied blush should enhance the shape of your face and flatter your bone structure. Learn the shape of your cheeks, so that you feel confident about where to apply colour. Smile at yourself in the mirror – the two cushiony areas that stand out are the 'apples'. Suck in your cheeks and feel the hollows and cheekbones.

For a natural flush of colour, use a soft pink or apricot, or a sheer stain or tint.

Dab blush on the apple of your cheek using a brush for powder (see right) and fingers or a sponge for other textures. Don't apply colour near the hairline or above the cheekbone, since you won't be able to blend it out.

If you're using a brush, make sure the head is not so large that you can't control where you're placing it. Sweep the brush over the product and tap or blow away any excess before applying.

Blend the colour from the apple upwards along the cheekbone, but don't take it down towards the nose or the hollow of the cheek. Lighten and soften all the edges, so that there is no line of colour and the blush fades seamlessly.

My secret It's easier to add colour than to remove it, so start with a little and build up the intensity. If you need more, apply at the apple and blend out.

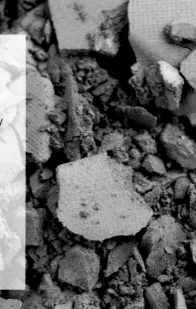

BRONZER APPLICATION

Big fat brushes can be difficult to control and make it easy to put on too much product. Apply powder bronzer with a smaller brush, tapping off the excess first. Crème or liquid bronzer should be applied with a sponge or your fingers and blended out.

Apply bronzer only where your face would naturally catch the sun – along the forehead, nose bridge, chin and cheekbones. Lightly apply bronzer in the middle of the cheek and blend out towards the hairline in one direction and towards the nose in the other, making sure you soften the edges well.

There's nothing worse than a bronzed face with a white neck and décolletage, so apply a light dusting of bronzer to the collarbone and the column of the neck.

When using bronzer to add warmth and shape to the face, apply it in the hollow of the cheekbones and on the temples.

My secret You can still wear blush and highlighter with bronzer, but apply tone-on-tone colours with subtlety – a golden highlighter will work better than white or silver-based highlighter.

Texture

Powder blush is available in endless shades and is easy to layer for deeper intensity. Those with a slight sheen bring a glow to the skin that is more flattering than flat matte textures. Today's formulations are ultra-fine and light, but powder blush will blend well only if your face has a dusting of translucent powder to create an even surface and ensure it won't stick and look patchy – take care that it doesn't crease in any fine lines. The soft velvety finish gives a polished, glamorous look that is hard to beat for night-time or winter looks.

Liquid stains, gel tints and crèmes create a natural-looking youthful blush that is ideal for daytime. They are easier to work than powder, as well as being more forgiving of mistakes. Tints and stains often come in a stick, tube or bottle with a brush or rollerball; all these work well. Don't be frightened by the bright colours – when blended on skin they produce a sheer wash of pinched-cheek colour. These formulations blend only on unpowdered or bare and moisturized skin, so make sure foundation has soaked in and hasn't dried to a powdery finish before you apply. Crèmes are the most moisturizing, making them ideal for dry or mature skin, while gels and stains work well on oilier skins as they are unlikely to slip. Wash your hands after application to prevent the pigment from staining.

Bronzer

Crème, liquid or powder bronzer can look fantastic, giving skin a lightly sunkissed glow, but it's easy to get wrong. The biggest mistake is to confuse bronzer with self-tan – you should never apply bronzer all over the face, as it will look like a mask: use it to highlight features or add a subtle glow in key areas.

Choose the colour carefully – bronzer with an orange or red base gets too close to an obvious fake tan, so look for a natural tan, which is more of a dirty bronze. If you can't find the right shade, go for a duo or trio bronzer that you can blend. Bronzers with too much shimmer can make you look very shiny and are ageing on mature skin. For a subtle glow, pick a bronzer containing soft pearl – not glitter – particles. If you're using bronzer to contour, choose a matte finish.

As with blush, don't apply powder bronzer onto moisturized skin, as the pigment sticks to the oils, making it hard to blend. Make sure your skin is dry or dust with fine translucent powder first. Bronzer can draw attention to blemishes and redness, so cover any imperfections with concealer before you apply.

Sculpting the cheekbones

Prominent cheekbones slim the face and suggest dignity – here's how to accentuate them. (A word of warning – if you have a round face, embrace it: faked cheekbones will look artificial.)

1 Use a deeper colour than on the apples of your cheeks, but not one too dark for your skin tone or it will look obvious – try beige or pale bronze on very pale skin, or deep bronze or honey on darker skin.

2 Using your fingers or a sponge for crème or a medium-sized brush for powder, apply a small amount of colour in the hollow underneath the cheekbones. Don't go all the way to the hairline or too low towards the jaw. Blend well, so there are no hard edges.

3 Apply dots of highlighter along the top of the cheekbone, just below and around the eye. Use your fingers or a brush to blend this out carefully. The different shades of blush should not overlap.

4 Balance the look by adding a touch of contour colour at the temples. A square or heavy jaw might need a touch of colour along the sides of the jaw.

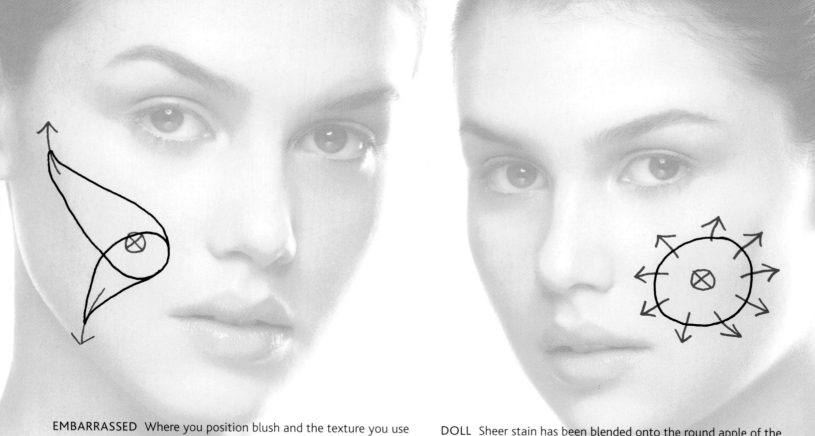

EMBARRASSED Where you position blush and the texture you use can create very different effects. Experiment to see what suits your face shape best. Here crème blush has been blended low down the cheek, fading softly towards the jaw, as though she's embarrassed.

DOLL Sheer stain has been blended onto the round apple of the cheek for a pretty, fresh, doll-like flush.

ELONGATED The cheekbone has been accentuated with subtle shading, using a slightly darker colour in the hollow beneath the bone and a fresher pink on the apple of the cheek, blended a little way along the cheekbone itself (see Sculpting the cheekbones on page 125).

RADIANT For a natural radiant blush, light-reflecting powder blush has been blended from the apple of the cheek along the cheekbone. This is the classic blush application that suits everyone (see page 124).

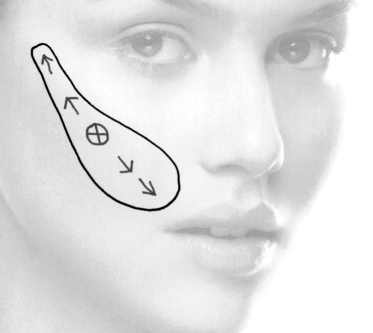

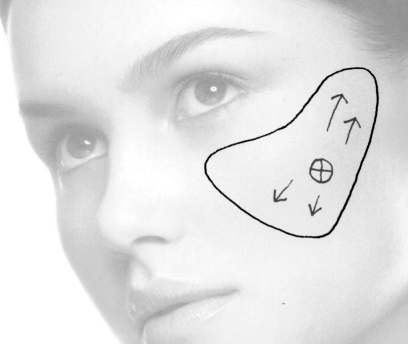

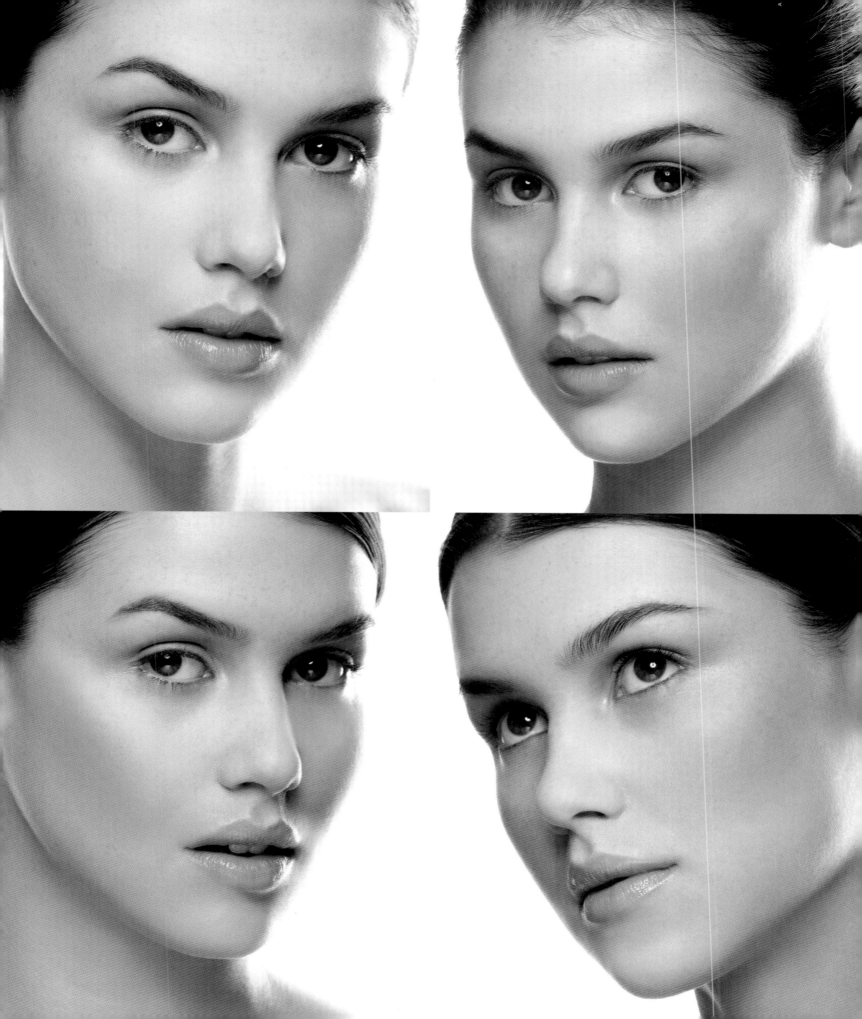

PERFECT POUT

Lip colour is one of the most fun and accessible areas of make-up, and also one of the most noticeable. From pretty and natural through classic and sophisticated to glamorous and vampish, how we make up our lips can change our mood in an instant.

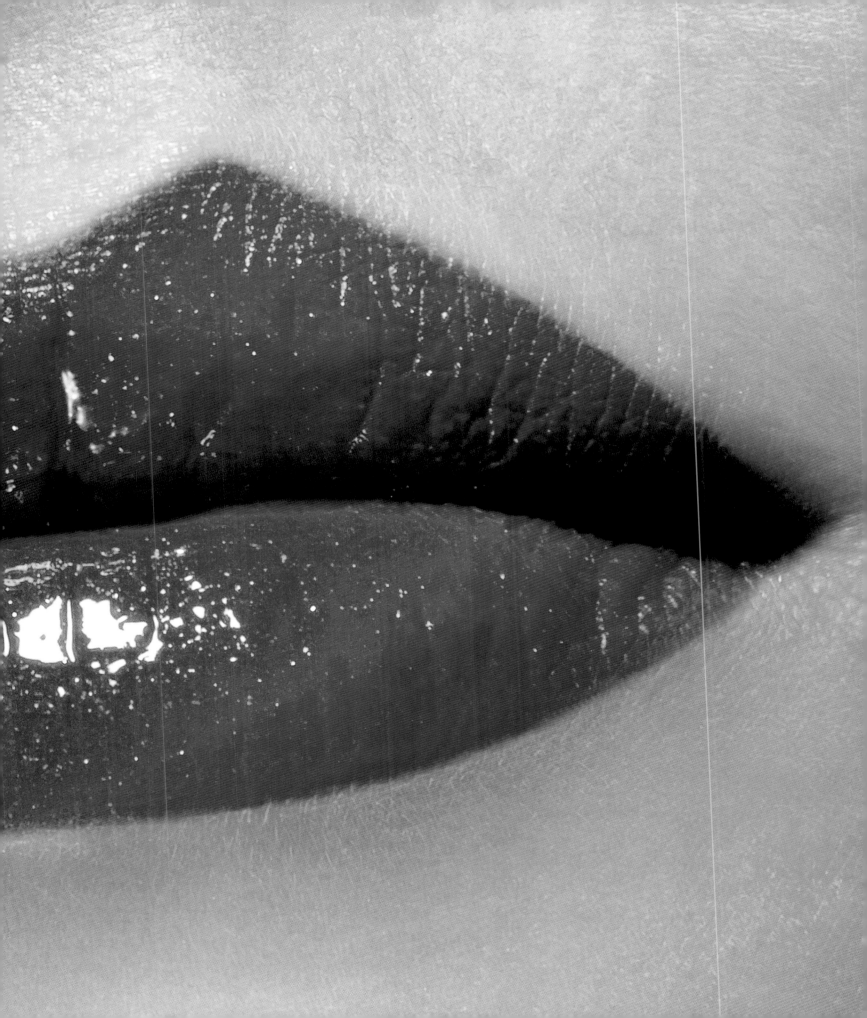

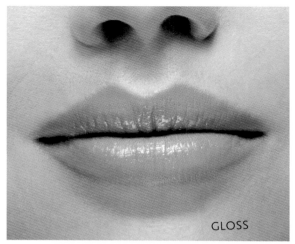
GLOSS

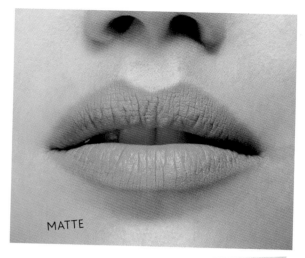
MATTE

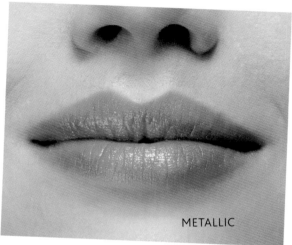
METALLIC

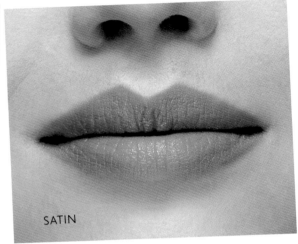
SATIN

finish

Natural or coloured, beautiful lips are full, pouting and sensuous – whether they're dramatic and matte, smooth and creamy, luscious and glossy or bee-stung and stained.

Texture

Lipsticks come in every texture imaginable – sheer, satin, metallic, frost, matte and high shine. Advanced formulations contain an array of moisturizing, hydrating, antioxidant, SPF, plumping, antifeathering and line-smoothing ingredients, so there's no excuse for a less-than-perfect pout. The finish you choose depends on the look you're going for, the time of year, and your age, skin tone and lip shape. Here are some pointers:

» Light tinted glosses with a silky rather than sticky texture are low-maintenance and youthful. Simply sweep gloss onto your lips with the wand or your finger, or line and fill in the lip with a matching pencil and apply gloss with a brush for a more defined look.

» Bright colours are more forgiving in a gloss finish than a matte one, which can look severe and ageing.

» Glossy, shiny and frosted finishes make lips look fuller than opaque, matte finishes.

» Lip stains look dark in their packaging but give the most natural wash of colour. Sweep the stain over each lip and press together to distribute evenly. Dab clear gloss onto the centre of the bottom lip to add some shine.

» Lipstick requires greater precision in application than glosses and stains, both of which can be worn without lipliner and are easy to reapply on the go.

» For daytime, a sheer, moisturizing lipstick is casual and flattering; a matte finish can seem heavy and unnatural in daylight.

» For evening, matte lipstick has a vintage appeal and gives intense colour with good staying power. Shimmering gloss also looks wonderful but will need to be reapplied.

» Matte lips look great in winter, but a natural sheen is lighter for summer.

Gloss gives a light shine to a base of lipliner or lipstick. A glossy finish makes a pout full and sexy.

Matte lipstick can't be beaten for a long-lasting no-shine finish, but choose a moisturizing formulation. Use matching lipliner and apply the lipstick with a brush for the greatest precision.

Metallic lipstick bounces light off the lips, giving a reflective shine that's great for a dramatic evening look.

Satin lipstick gives a semi-sheer semi-matte finish. It has a hydrating formula and is super-flattering for everyday wear.

Colour

Cooler blue-based colours tend to suit pink-toned skin, while warmer orange-based shades are more flattering on yellow-based complexions. Hair colour doesn't affect what colour will suit you and the best advice is to try, try, try until you find your favourite shades. If you can't try the lipstick directly on your lips – most cosmetics counters do provide alcohol wipes for hygiene – try it on your fingertip, look in a mirror and hold your finger up next to your mouth. Here are some pointers:

» Bare or neutral colours look fantastic on everyone, especially for day.

» Pinks warm up pale or older skin.

» Golden red colours are lovely on tanned or dark complexions.

» Pale or glossy lipsticks make thin lips look fuller.

» Full lips can get away with dark or matte shades.

» Dark lipstick, especially harsh reds and chocolate browns, is more ageing than any other make-up choice.

» When using a lip pencil for outlining only, choose a neutral colour that blends with your skin tone. If you match your lipliner to your lipstick, fill in the entire lip area, otherwise it will look unnatural as the lipstick wears off.

'When shopping for the perfect colour, try lipstick on your fingertip – the skin there is most similar in colour and texture to your lips and will give a fairly close representation of the effect.'

LIP CARE

Lips are one of the few areas of the body that don't have sweat glands, so the skin dries out more easily. No lipstick or gloss looks good on chapped lips and some matte lipsticks dry lips even more, while many plumpers contain ingredients that overstimulate and sting. Keep lips smooth and moisturized with a balm containing natural oils, such as beeswax, and SPF. If you have chapped lips, apply balm and after a few minutes massage gently with a soft toothbrush or flannel. Alternatively, exfoliate gently with a lip polish or scrub. Even if you don't wear any other make-up, protect your lips by wearing a tinted balm or moisturizing gloss.

Bright lips

Coral, tangerine and cherry lipsticks are difficult to wear, but with the right approach they can be sophisticated and bring out the golden tones in skin.

» Bright oranges look great on women with medium to dark complexions – those with very fair skin or red hair should give them a miss.

» A gloss finish makes these colours more wearable, but if you want a strong matte look, use a nude lipliner to stop colour running.

» Keep the rest of your make-up quiet, with nude eyes and natural lightly bronzed cheeks – the wrong blush can clash with the lips.

Nude lips

Pale, glossy lips look full and healthy. They are flattering for most women, night or day, and balance the effect when you wear dramatic eye make-up.

» Cover your natural lip colour using a little foundation in a slightly darker shade – the one you wear when you're tanned is ideal.

» Apply moisturizing lip balm on top of the foundation – if you apply it first, the oils will prevent the foundation from sinking in properly.

» Either apply a little clear gloss on top of the balm, or choose a natural beige, pink or taupe lipstick with a creamy texture – lips should be plumped with a slight shine but not a mirror gloss.

» Layer coloured gloss over sheer brown or beige lipstick for a modern, edgy depth of colour.

red lips

For the elegant glamour of 1950s Hollywood, red lips never go out of style, but precision is essential. Choose a lipstick that suits your colouring – deep, plummy reds look fantastic on dark skin, cool blue-based reds suit pink-toned and pale skin, while orange-based reds are less draining on a warmer complexion (but make sure it doesn't accentuate any redness in your cheeks).

1 Prepare your lips well (see page 131). Dab foundation around the lip area and over the lip itself. This tones down any redness and ensures the line of the lips will be sharp and defined.

2 Use a matching waxy lipliner to prevent any bleed around the lips. Spend time drawing the outline, making sure the lips are completely symmetrical and the bow is even. An uneven top lip shows up with red lipstick more than any other colour. Start at the V of the Cupid's bow and take the liner right into the corners.

3 Fill in the lip with the pencil to hold the lipstick in place and make it last longer. Go over the pencil colour with a lip brush, working it into any creases.

4 Paint on the lipstick using a lip brush for precision, starting in one corner and working inwards. Use the tip of the brush for the edges and the flat of the brush for larger areas. Blot with a tissue and apply another coat.

5 Add a dab of gloss in a clear or slightly lighter shade at the centre of the lower lip and press your lips together to give an illusion of fullness.

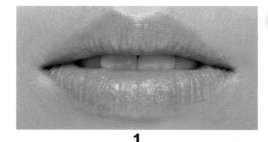

1

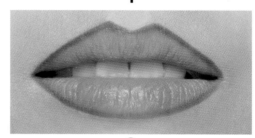

2

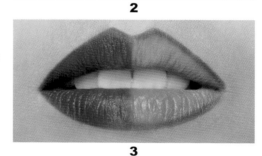

3

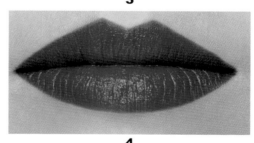

4

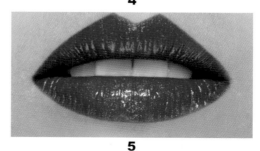

5

TOP TIPS

Red lips spell grown-up glamour and should be worn with confidence.

» Hair colour is irrelevant when choosing the right shade of red – it's skin tone that counts. Pink tones are best suited to cooler 'blue reds', while darker, Mediterranean and Asian skins are better suited to 'orange reds'.

» Red lips will be the focus, so keep the rest of your make-up minimal.

» A red-tinted lipgloss will give a more subtle effect.

» Try not to touch your mouth so you don't risk smudging the lipstick. Matte finishes are more resistant to smudging than gloss.

My secret Avoid picking up lipstick colour on your gloss wand by dabbing gloss onto your finger then applying it to your lower lip. Press lips together a few times to distribute evenly.

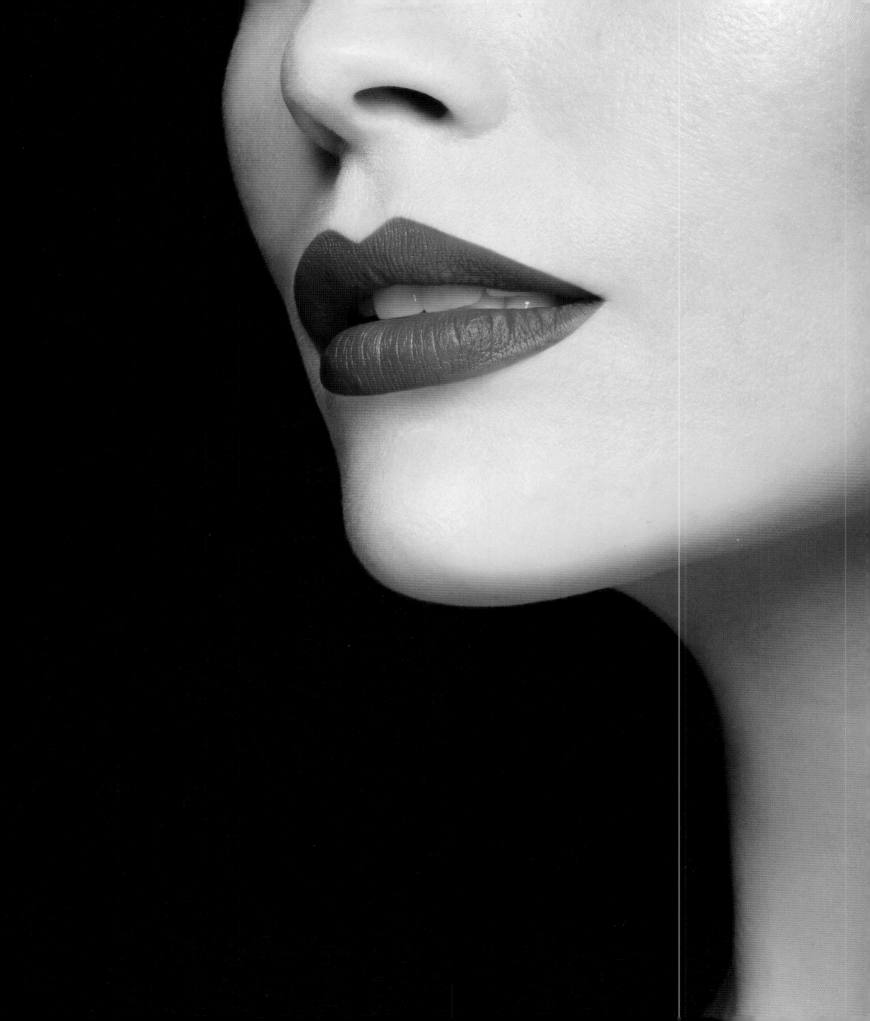

lip shape

Lip shape affects not only how you apply lipstick but also the colours you should wear. For a perfect pout, lips should be completely symmetrical – the depth of the fattest part of the upper lip should be equal to that of the lower lip, and the left and right halves, from the centre of the Cupid's bow to the centre of the bottom lip, should be mirror images of each other (see right). Lip pencil is an invaluable tool in achieving perfect symmetry, enabling you to 'correct' any irregularities by drawing a hair's breadth inside or outside the lip line.

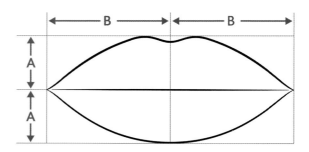

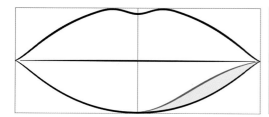

If your lip shape is slightly wonky, draw just outside the natural lip line to correct the shape and achieve perfect symmetry.

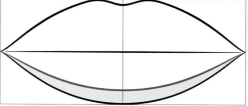

If your lower lip is thinner than your upper lip, add depth to the lower lip by drawing just outside the natural lip line.

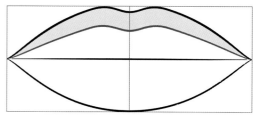

If your lower lip is fuller than your top lip, draw just outside the upper lip line to create fullness, taking extra care when drawing the Cupid's bow. A touch of highlighter above the upper lip will add to the illusion.

HOW TO OUTLINE YOUR LIPS

- Apply a little foundation around the lip area before you start to provide a neutral base.

- Draw the outline with pencil to ensure total symmetry, starting at the central V of the Cupid's bow and drawing to each corner with short, feathery strokes. A common mistake is to leave a gap here, or to draw too wide.

- If you make a mistake, use a cotton bud dipped in a little make-up remover to push the smudge inwards onto the lip, rather than wiping it away from the mouth onto the face.

- Once you're happy with the outline, fill in the whole lip with pencil and go over the colour with a brush to make sure it's completely even – this will make lipstick stay on longer. Creamy liners are easier to work with a brush.

- Apply lipstick with a lip brush – this gives greater precision than applying it directly from the tube.

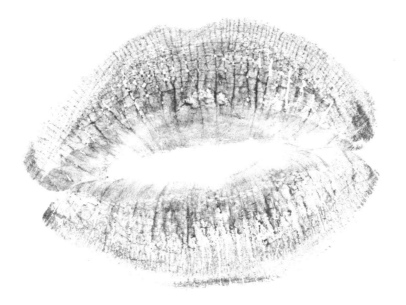

Thin lips

» Use sheer, shimmery shades – dark colours make a mouth look severe, while lighter shades make lips look fuller.

» Using a lipliner that matches your lipstick, accentuate your lips by drawing on the outer edge of your lip line.

» For a fuller pout, add a dot of shimmering gloss at the centre of the lower lip and blend it out by pressing your lips together.

» Plump up your pout by wearing a lip plumper alone or under lipstick.

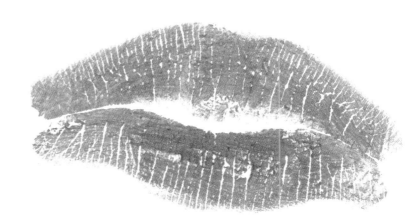

Overfull lips

» Darker colours and matte textures make lips seem smaller. Avoid very pale shades or shimmery textures as they can make lips seem fuller.

» Use a neutral lipliner to draw just inside your lip line. Alternatively, don't use lipliner but apply lipstick with a brush, placing the colour at the centre of your lips and blending it out.

» If the bottom lip is larger than the top, use lipliner on the top but not on the bottom, and they will seem to match more evenly.

Feathery lines

» Use a lipliner, the waxier the better – it forms a barrier that helps lipstick stay on the lip.

» The brighter the lipstick, the more obvious the bleed will be, so use a neutral lipliner, even if you then choose to fill in the shape with a brighter lipstick.

» Blot with a tissue after application. Apply a little translucent powder around the lip to help seal in colour.

TOP TEN LIP LOOKS

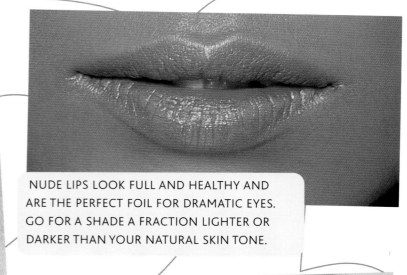

NUDE LIPS LOOK FULL AND HEALTHY AND
ARE THE PERFECT FOIL FOR DRAMATIC EYES.
GO FOR A SHADE A FRACTION LIGHTER OR
DARKER THAN YOUR NATURAL SKIN TONE.

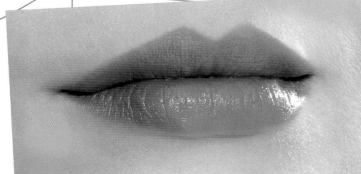

LIP STAIN GIVES SHEER LONG-LASTING
NATURAL COLOUR. ADD A TOUCH OF GLOSS
OR LAYER UNDER LIPSTICK FOR ADDED DEPTH.

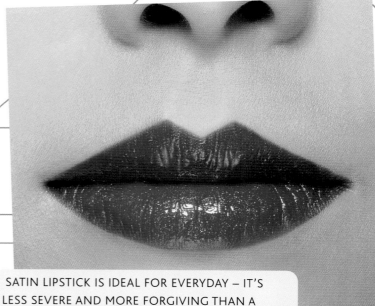

SATIN LIPSTICK IS IDEAL FOR EVERYDAY – IT'S
LESS SEVERE AND MORE FORGIVING THAN A
MATTE FINISH AND MORE SUBTLE THAN GLOSS.

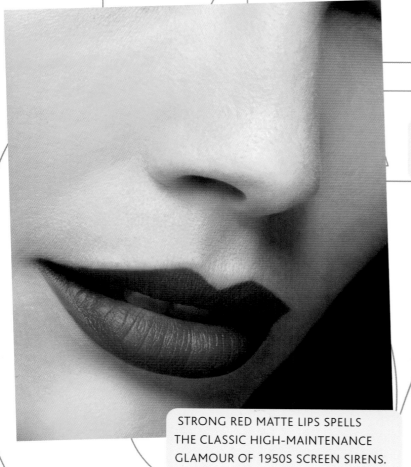

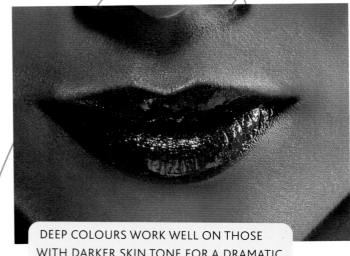

STRONG RED MATTE LIPS SPELLS
THE CLASSIC HIGH-MAINTENANCE
GLAMOUR OF 1950S SCREEN SIRENS.

DEEP COLOURS WORK WELL ON THOSE
WITH DARKER SKIN TONE FOR A DRAMATIC
NIGHT-TIME LOOK. BALANCE WITH
STRONG WELL-DEFINED BROWS.

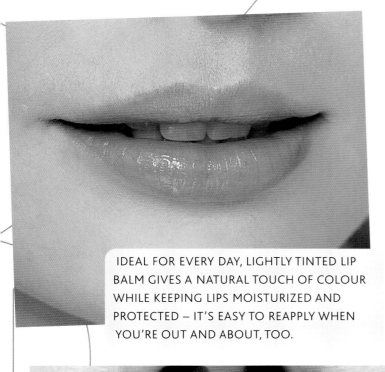

IDEAL FOR EVERY DAY, LIGHTLY TINTED LIP BALM GIVES A NATURAL TOUCH OF COLOUR WHILE KEEPING LIPS MOISTURIZED AND PROTECTED – IT'S EASY TO REAPPLY WHEN YOU'RE OUT AND ABOUT, TOO.

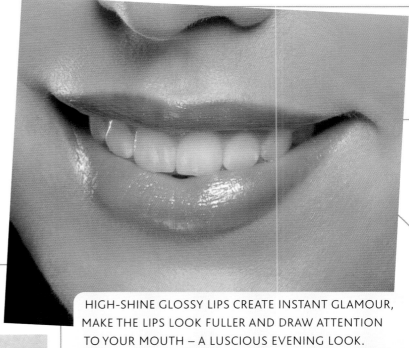

HIGH-SHINE GLOSSY LIPS CREATE INSTANT GLAMOUR, MAKE THE LIPS LOOK FULLER AND DRAW ATTENTION TO YOUR MOUTH – A LUSCIOUS EVENING LOOK.

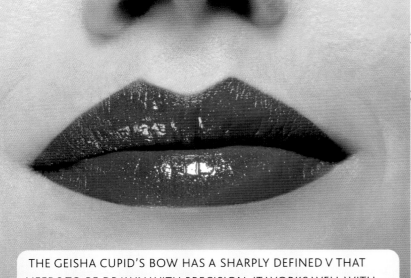

THE GEISHA CUPID'S BOW HAS A SHARPLY DEFINED V THAT NEEDS TO BE DRAWN WITH PRECISION. IT WORKS WELL WITH STRONG, BRIGHT COLOURS IN GLOSS OR MATTE.

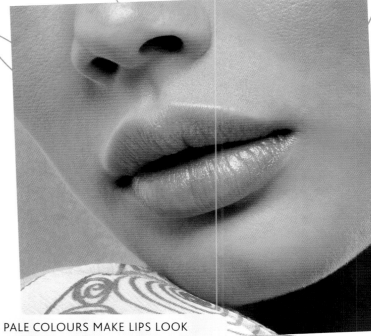

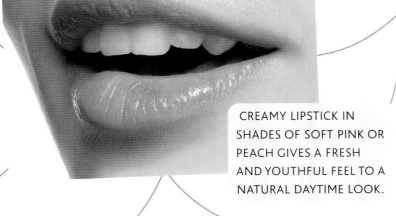

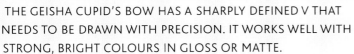

CREAMY LIPSTICK IN SHADES OF SOFT PINK OR PEACH GIVES A FRESH AND YOUTHFUL FEEL TO A NATURAL DAYTIME LOOK.

PALE COLOURS MAKE LIPS LOOK FULLER. ADD A TOUCH OF HIGHLIGHTER ABOVE THE CUPID'S BOW AND DRAW JUST OUTSIDE THE NATURAL LIP LINE. A DAB OF GLOSS AT THE CENTRE OF THE LOWER LIP WILL ACCENTUATE YOUR POUT.

NEAT NAILS

From a barely there French manicure, to classic red, to dramatic chocolate and navy, to fashion-forward neons and metallics, immaculately manicured nails always give a groomed and polished impression.

Available in a rainbow of colours – from natural beiges and pale pinks, through every imaginable shade of red, to statement colours such as acid yellow, grey and black – nail varnishes also come in plain, glitter, pearlized and metallic finishes. Think of your nails as an accessory and experiment with different looks. Bear in mind that pale, nude colours are easier to apply and lower maintenance than dark colours, which show up smudges and chips more readily and look good only when they're gleaming. Soft, natural colours can be worn with most shades of lipstick without risk of them clashing.

As a rule, you get what you pay for and the more expensive varnishes tend to go on more evenly, have a more intense colour and last longer without chipping. To prolong their life, screw the lid on tightly and store in a cool, dark place.

My secret If you are wearing a really wild colour on your nails, keep the other elements of your look fairly neutral.

Mix or match?

Fashions come and go, so it's up to you whether you match your fingers to your toes, and your nails to your lipstick. Here are some pointers:

» Make sure your nail varnish doesn't clash with your lipstick.

» In general, it is more flattering to have lighter fingernails and darker toes.

» Different shades within the same colour family look elegant. Try beige or tan on fingers and a bronze or warm coffee on toes, or try soft pink on fingers with a stronger pink on toes.

» Contrasting shades that complement each other because they are both warm- or cool-based can work well. A shimmering white on the fingers looks great with blood-red toes, for example.

» Never mix orange and pink or apricot and red.

TOP TIPS FOR HEALTHY NAILS

» Moisturize hands and feet regularly and use cuticle oil to condition the skin around the nails. Wear rubber gloves for housework and don't wear ill-fitting shoes.

» Buffing smooths ridges, making the nail surface shine and varnish go on more evenly. Don't buff nails more than every couple of weeks, or you may weaken the nail bed.

» Always apply base coat under varnish. It provides a surface for the varnish to adhere to and prevents it from staining the nail.

» Always apply top coat – it helps the varnish to last longer and gives a mirror-like shine. Fast-drying top coat speeds up the drying process.

» Chipped nails look awful and are more noticeable on dark varnish. Don't pick at it, as this weakens the nail – take it off using nail varnish remover.

» False nails ruin the condition of natural nails – don't be tempted.

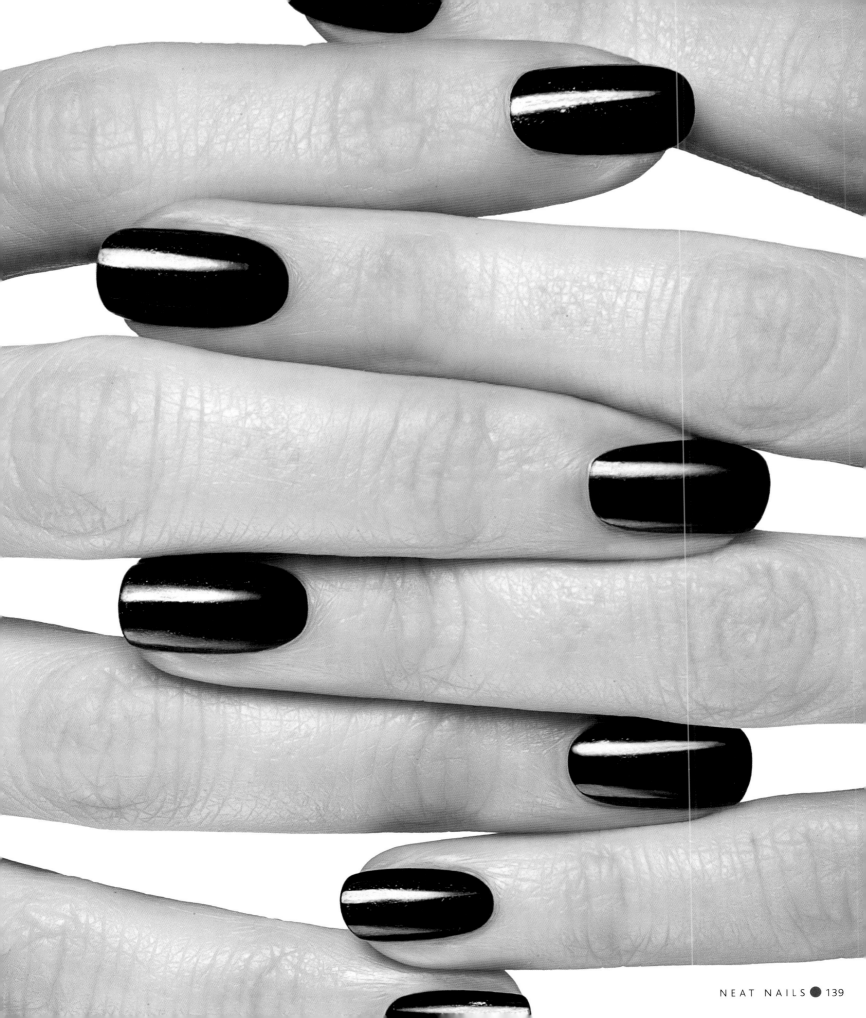

DIY manicure or pedicure

With nail bars on every high street, professional manicures and pedicures need no longer be reserved for special occasions. Yet with a little time and practice, it's not hard to keep your hands, feet and nails healthy, tidy and polished.

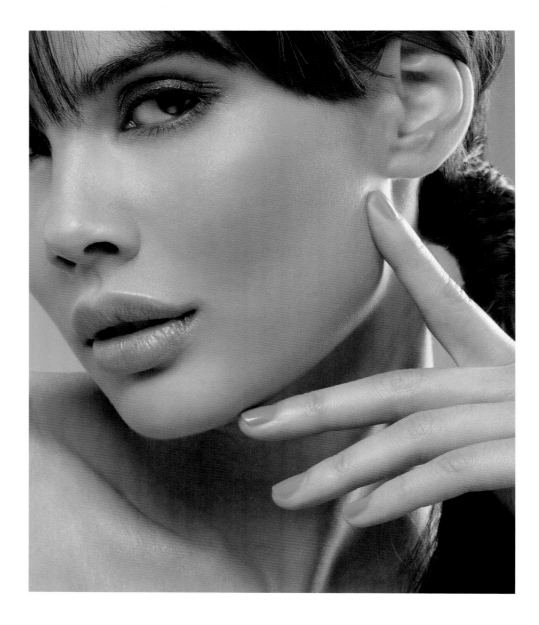

TOOL KIT

» NAILBRUSH – for scrubbing nails clean.

» NAIL CLIPPERS – for cutting toenails straight across.

» SHARP NAIL SCISSORS WITH CURVED EDGES – for cutting fingernails.

» CUTICLE REMOVER – a cream to remove dead skin from the cuticle area.

» NAIL STONE – a pen-shaped pumice for removing dead skin from the surface.

» CUTICLE NIPPERS WITH POINTED TIPS – for trimming hangnails.

» WOODEN OR PLASTIC ORANGE STICK – for gently pushing back the cuticles.

» NAIL BUFFER – for smoothing and shining the nail surface

» EMERY BOARD – for filing the edges of nails smooth.

» HAND/FOOT CREAM – for moisturizing and protecting (make sure hand cream contains SPF).

» CUTICLE CREAM – for softening the cuticles and preventing hangnails.

» NAIL/CUTICLE OIL – sweet almond oil and vitamin E to condition the nail bed and cuticle.

» CONDITIONING BASE COAT – to protect the nail and prevent it from becoming stained, and to provide a surface for the varnish to adhere to.

» TOP COAT – for a fast-drying, shiny, hard finish that helps to prevent varnish from chipping.

» ACETONE-FREE NAIL VARNISH REMOVER – to gently remove all traces of varnish without stripping the nails of moisture.

» FOAM TOE SEPARATOR – for holding the toes apart to avoid smudging while varnishing toenails.

How to be your own nail technician

1 Wipe off old varnish with a cotton pad moistened with nail varnish remover. Wash your hands thoroughly and scrub the nails with a nailbrush.

2 If necessary, trim the nails using sharp curved nail scissors for fingernails and clippers for toenails (always cut toenails straight across to prevent ingrown nails). Shorter nails look smarter, especially when painted in dark colours.

3 Use the emery board to file the nails, working in one direction only – don't saw back and forth. Create a gentle curve at the edges, so the nails are slightly squared off with rounded corners.

4 Gently buff the nails, sweeping the buffer across the nail bed to smooth any ridges and make the surface shine.

5 If necessary, apply cuticle remover following the pack instructions, or apply a little softening cuticle cream.

6 Using an orange stick, gently push back the cuticles from the nail to reveal a neat half-moon shape at the root. Carefully trim any hangnails with cuticle nippers.

7 Gently rub the nail with a nail stone to remove any dead skin, focusing on the edges closest to the cuticles.

8 Rinse and dry well. Then massage oil into the nails and cuticles and apply hand or foot cream.

TOP TIP

For smooth, soft feet, use a hard-skin remover once a week and buff your heels and soles with a foot file or pumice. Massage with moisturizing foot cream.

'Use a moisturizing hand cream with SPF. Keep a tube in your handbag, by your desk, by your bed and by the sink – and reapply it regularly.'

The perfect polish

1 Prepare the nails as described (see left). Wipe a cotton pad moistened with nail varnish remover over the nails to remove any trace of nail oil. Separate toes with foam separators or balls of cotton wool.

2 Apply base coat to each nail, being careful not to get it on the cuticles, as it will make them hard.

3 Starting a hair's breadth away from the cuticle, apply the first coat of varnish. Make one stroke down the centre of the nail first, then fill in the strips on either side. Once each nail has been painted, apply the second coat.

4 Apply a coat of fast-drying top coat and leave to dry. The varnish will be touch dry in around half an hour, but be careful with your hands and don't put on shoes for an hour.

TOP TIP

If you make a mistake, dip a cotton bud into nail varnish remover and wipe it away.

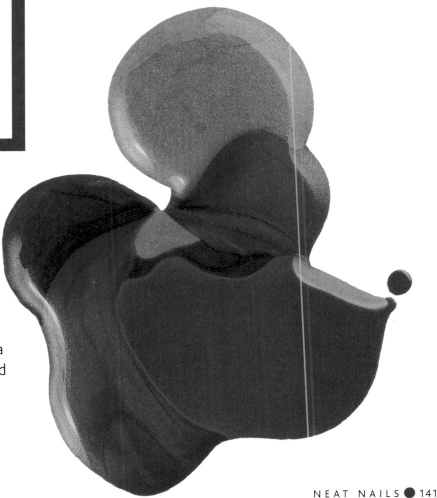

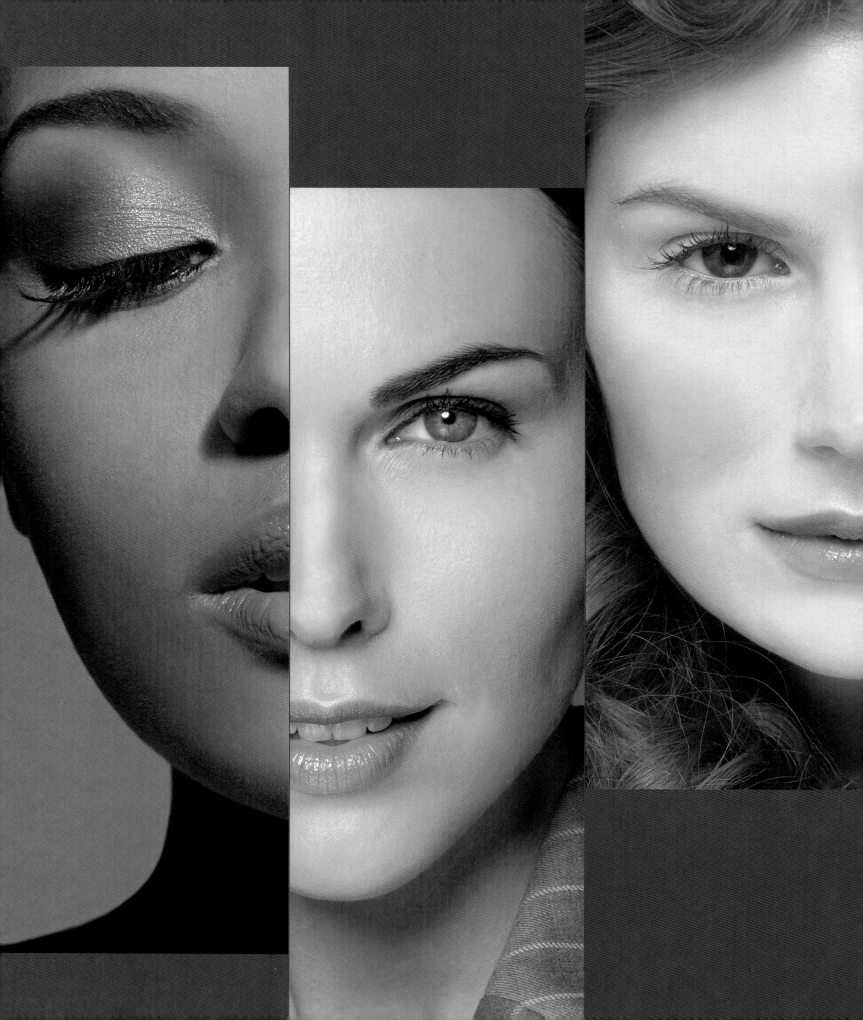

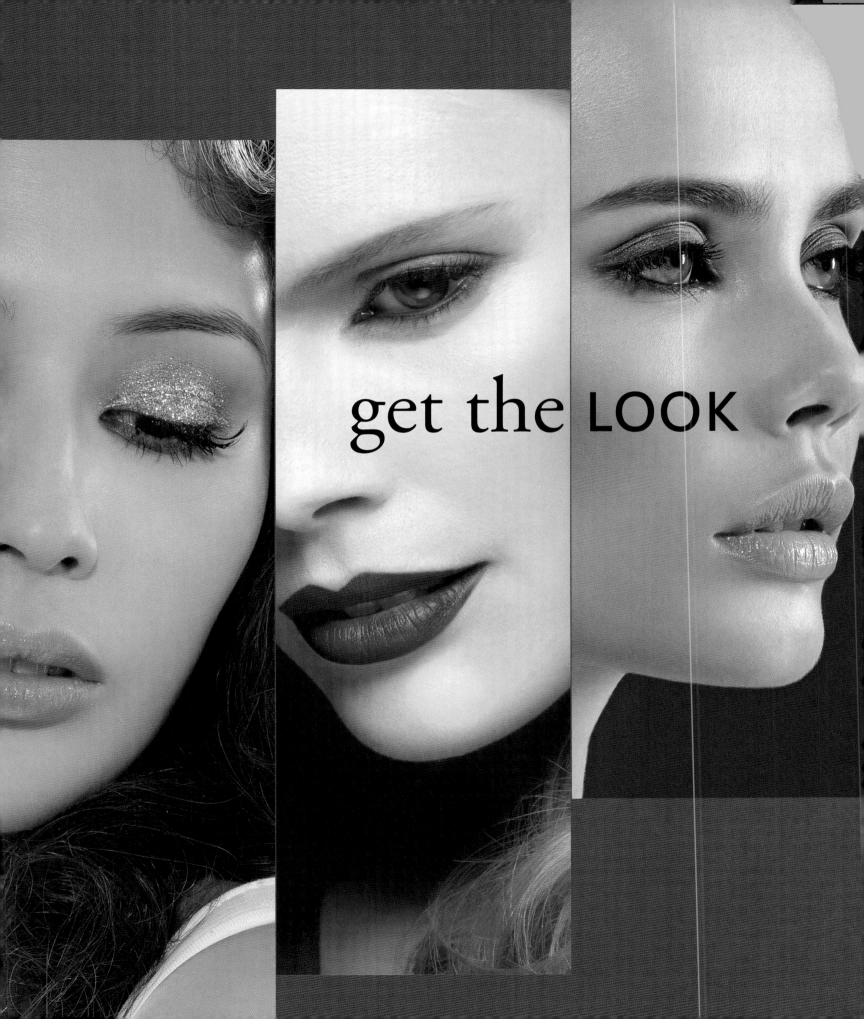

get the LOOK

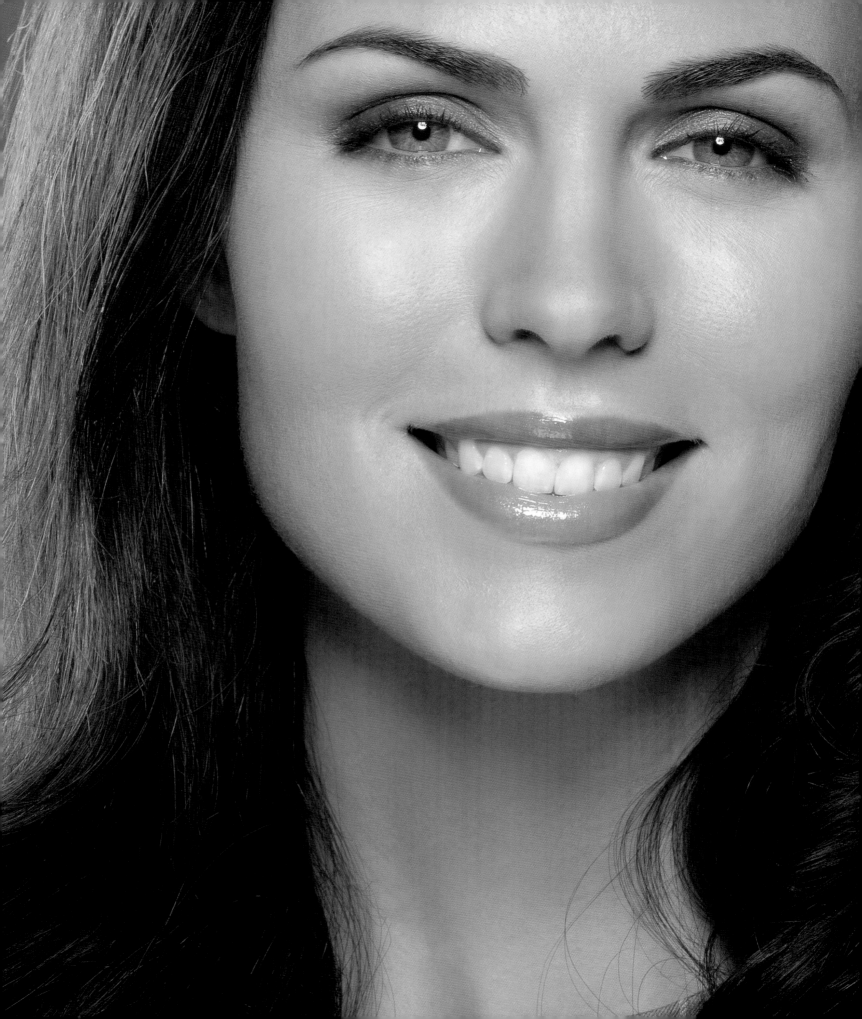

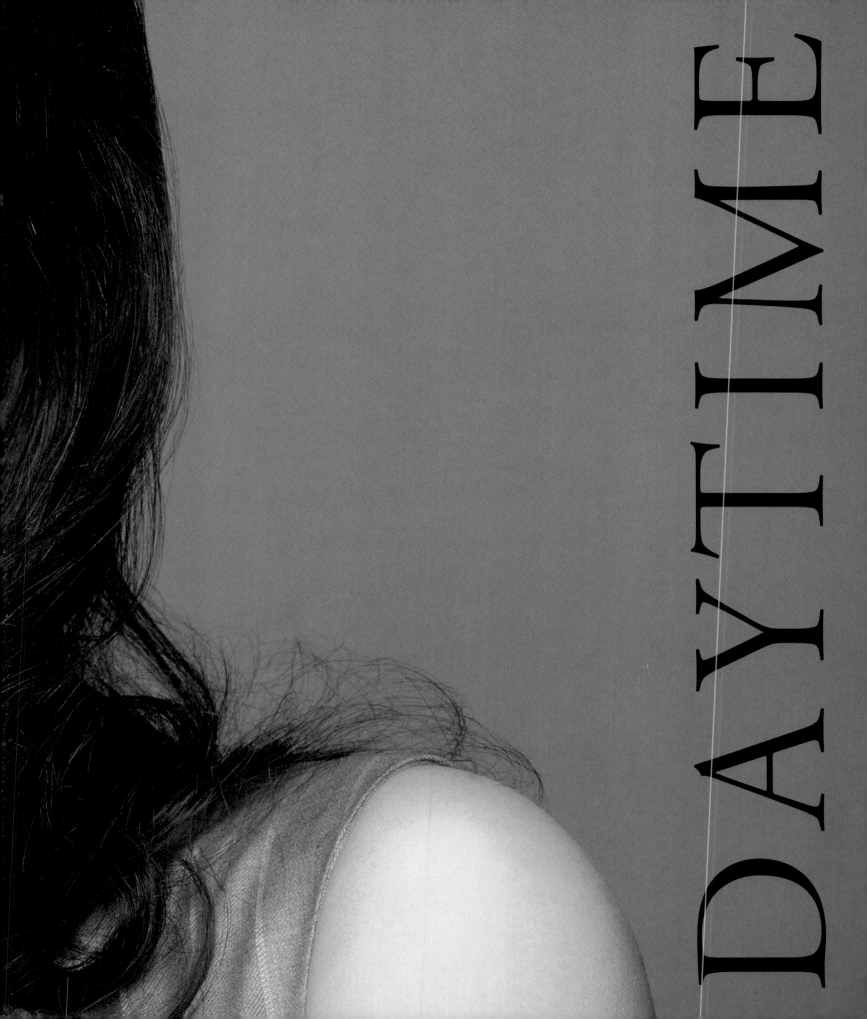

DAYTIME

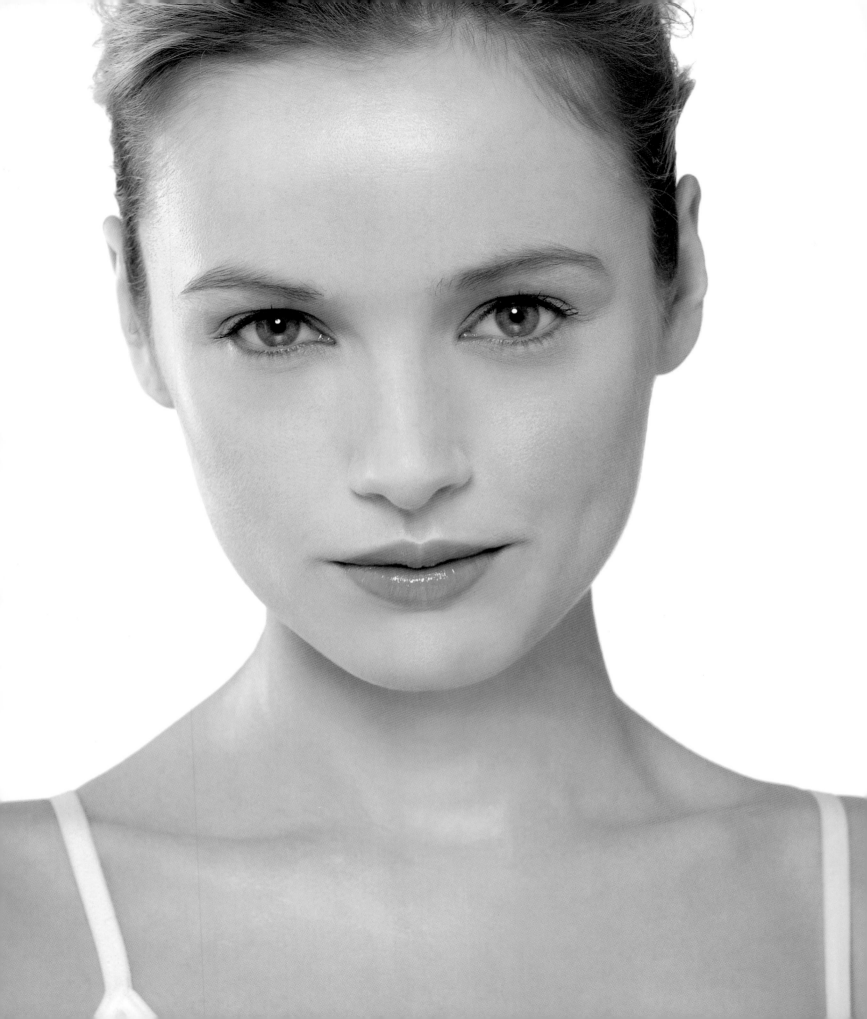

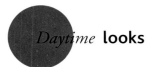

everyday gorgeous

I call this subtle type of make-up 'stealth make-up', as it ensures you look fabulous but not at all 'made up'. The effect is tidy, polished and groomed, with neat brows, curled lashes and subtly defined eyes. Skin is smooth, hydrated and natural – neither too dewy nor too matte. This is wearable everyday make-up that can take you anywhere, but while it seems as if you're hardly wearing any, the barely-there look requires careful application.

porcelain

Pale colours are the most flattering for a barely-there daytime look, as stronger colours will provide too much contrast. Creams, pearls and oysters with a slight sheen work well for eyes, with sheer or slightly glossy nude or pale pink shades for lips.

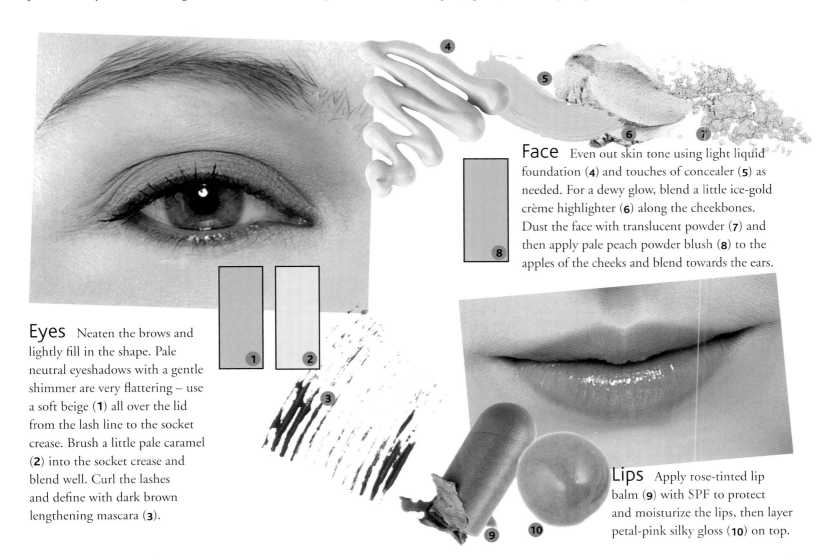

Face Even out skin tone using light liquid foundation (**4**) and touches of concealer (**5**) as needed. For a dewy glow, blend a little ice-gold crème highlighter (**6**) along the cheekbones. Dust the face with translucent powder (**7**) and then apply pale peach powder blush (**8**) to the apples of the cheeks and blend towards the ears.

Eyes Neaten the brows and lightly fill in the shape. Pale neutral eyeshadows with a gentle shimmer are very flattering – use a soft beige (**1**) all over the lid from the lash line to the socket crease. Brush a little pale caramel (**2**) into the socket crease and blend well. Curl the lashes and define with dark brown lengthening mascara (**3**).

Lips Apply rose-tinted lip balm (**9**) with SPF to protect and moisturize the lips, then layer petal-pink silky gloss (**10**) on top.

fair

A blend of fresh pink and soft pinky-beige blush gives fair skin a natural flush, which makes the face look healthy and youthful. Eyeshadow in pink-based shades of beige or taupe with a deeper brown for definition tends to be more flattering than yellow-based shades. Matte finishes or those with a slight shimmer work equally well. Lips can be nude, soft pink or warm brown.

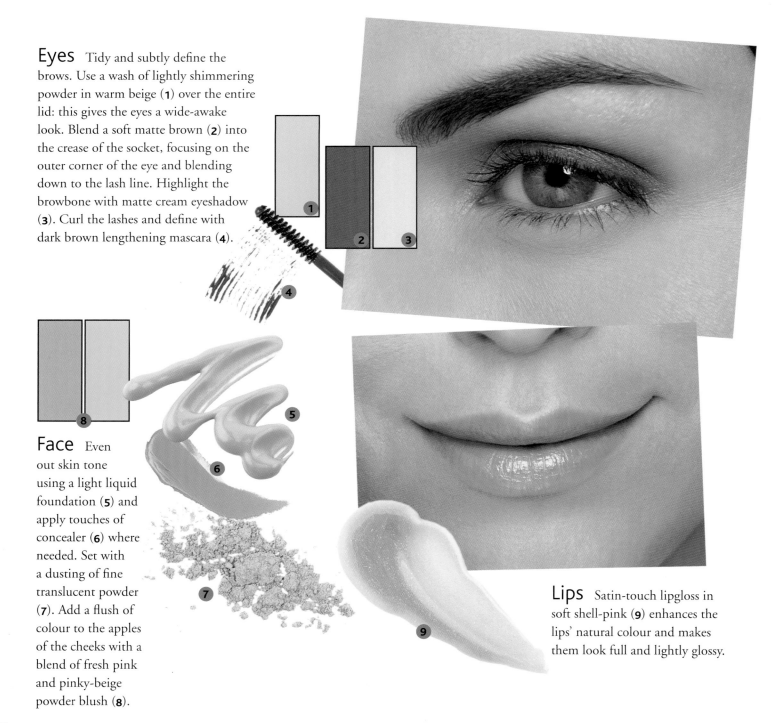

Eyes Tidy and subtly define the brows. Use a wash of lightly shimmering powder in warm beige (**1**) over the entire lid: this gives the eyes a wide-awake look. Blend a soft matte brown (**2**) into the crease of the socket, focusing on the outer corner of the eye and blending down to the lash line. Highlight the browbone with matte cream eyeshadow (**3**). Curl the lashes and define with dark brown lengthening mascara (**4**).

Face Even out skin tone using a light liquid foundation (**5**) and apply touches of concealer (**6**) where needed. Set with a dusting of fine translucent powder (**7**). Add a flush of colour to the apples of the cheeks with a blend of fresh pink and pinky-beige powder blush (**8**).

Lips Satin-touch lipgloss in soft shell-pink (**9**) enhances the lips' natural colour and makes them look full and lightly glossy.

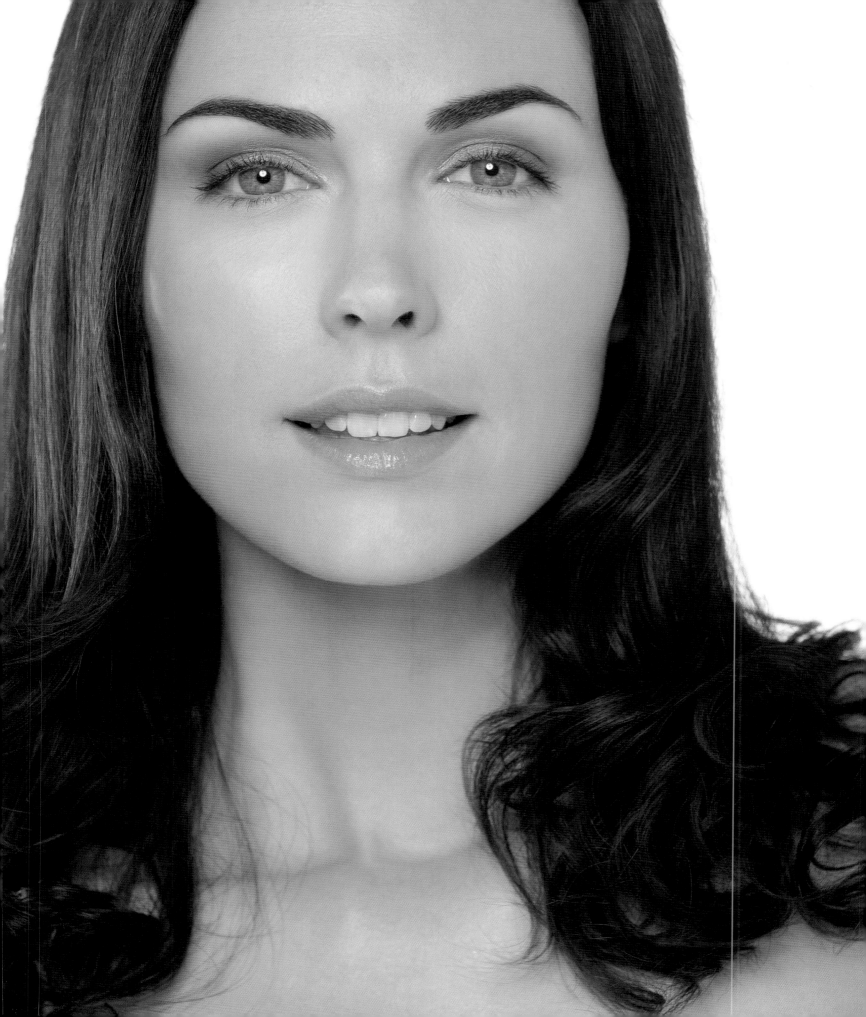

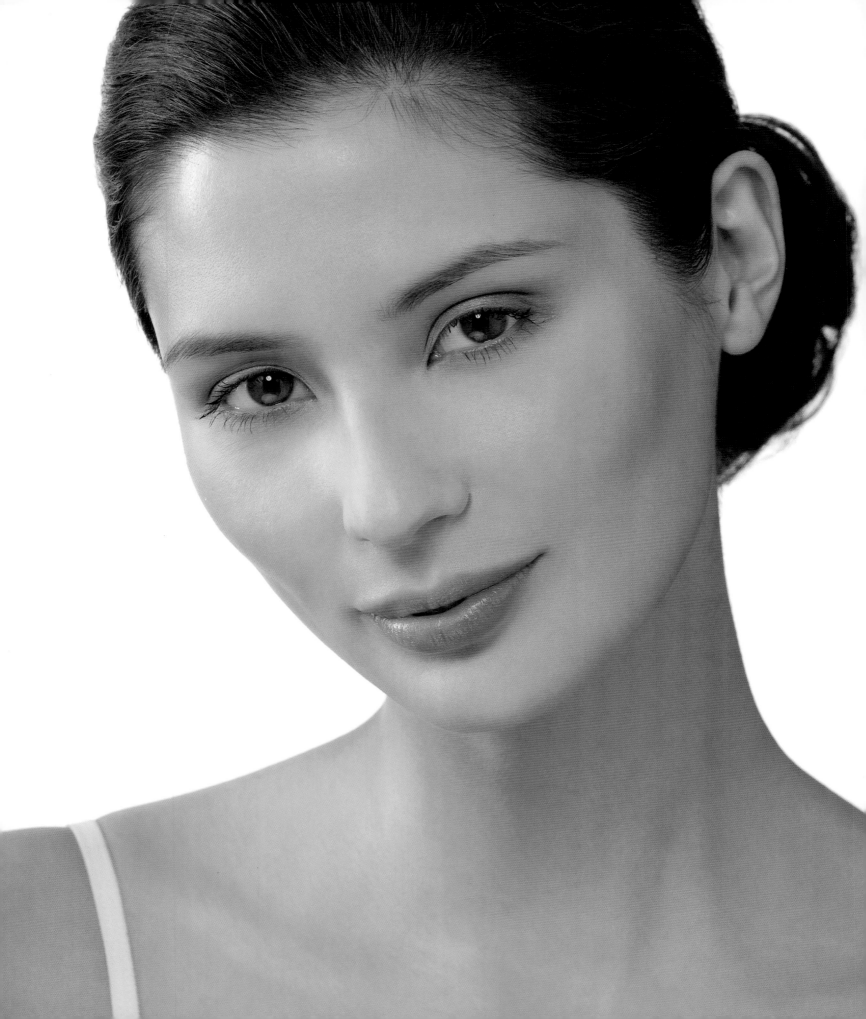

olive

Eyeshadows with yellow or orange undertones work best on olive skin. Go for pale neutrals in buttery creams, gold or peachy beige and soft browns. Nude, pale peach or sheer brown colours are very flattering on lips, while shades of pinky peach and warm beige give a natural blush.

Eyes Groom and define the brows, then subtly define the eyes with a blend of lightly shimmering beige gold and mushroomy brown powder eyeshadows. Apply a wash of beige gold (**1**) over the entire lid, then intensify the colour at the socket and outer corner of the eye with the darker shade (**2**), blending well. Curl the lashes and apply black lengthening mascara (**3**).

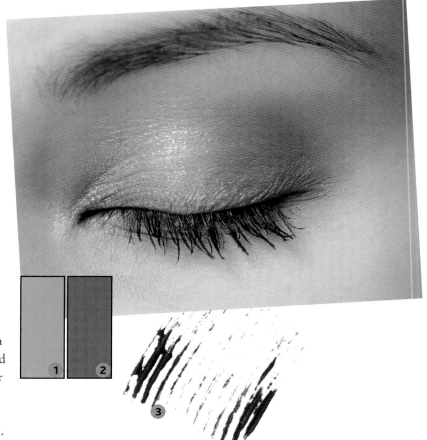

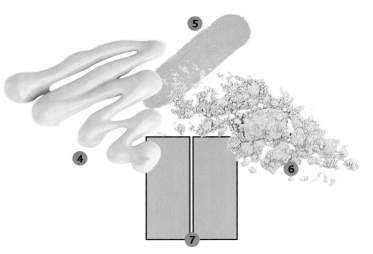

Face Even out skin tone using either a light liquid foundation (**4**) or a mineral foundation if your skin is prone to oiliness. Hide any blemishes with dabs of concealer (**5**). If you've used liquid foundation, set with a light dusting of translucent powder (**6**), then give the apples of the cheeks a natural flush using a blend of soft peach and sandy-beige powder blush (**7**).

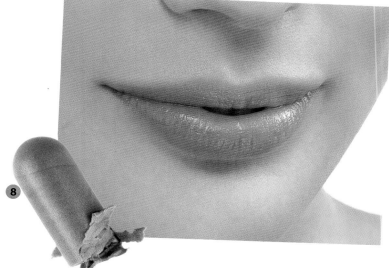

Lips Keep lips moisturized and protected with rose-tinted lip balm with SPF (**8**), which gives a light sheen of natural colour.

deep

Eyeshadows in chocolate brown, coffee, praline and taupe work best for a no-make-up look on deep skin tones, while lips look natural in sheer apricot or soft brown shades. A gentle sweep of bronzing powder is all that's needed to bring a little extra colour to the cheeks.

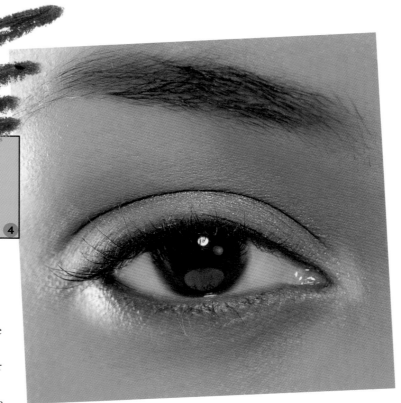

Face Even out skin tone with a light liquid foundation (**6**) or a mineral foundation if your skin is prone to oiliness. Hide any blemishes or discoloration with touches of concealer (**7**). If you've used liquid foundation, set with a light dusting of translucent powder (**8**), then brush a sweep of bronzing powder (**9**) onto the cheeks.

Eyes Shape and define the brows, then draw along the upper lash line and just under the lower lashes with earthy-brown eyeliner pencil (**1**). Use a smudger to soften the line, blending outwards at the outer corner. Apply a wash of lightly shimmering mid-brown eyeshadow (**2**) over the lid, then intensify the colour at the socket and outer corner with matte dark brown shadow (**3**). Add a touch of light-reflecting mocha eyeshadow (**4**) to highlight the browbone. Curl the lashes and apply black lengthening mascara (**5**).

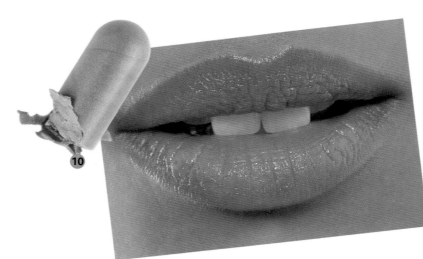
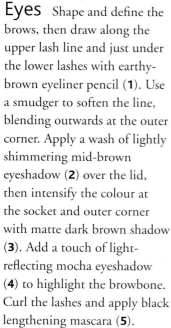

Lips Give lips a light sheen of natural colour with moisturizing apricot-tinted lip balm (**10**) with SPF to protect the lips and keep them luscious and soft.

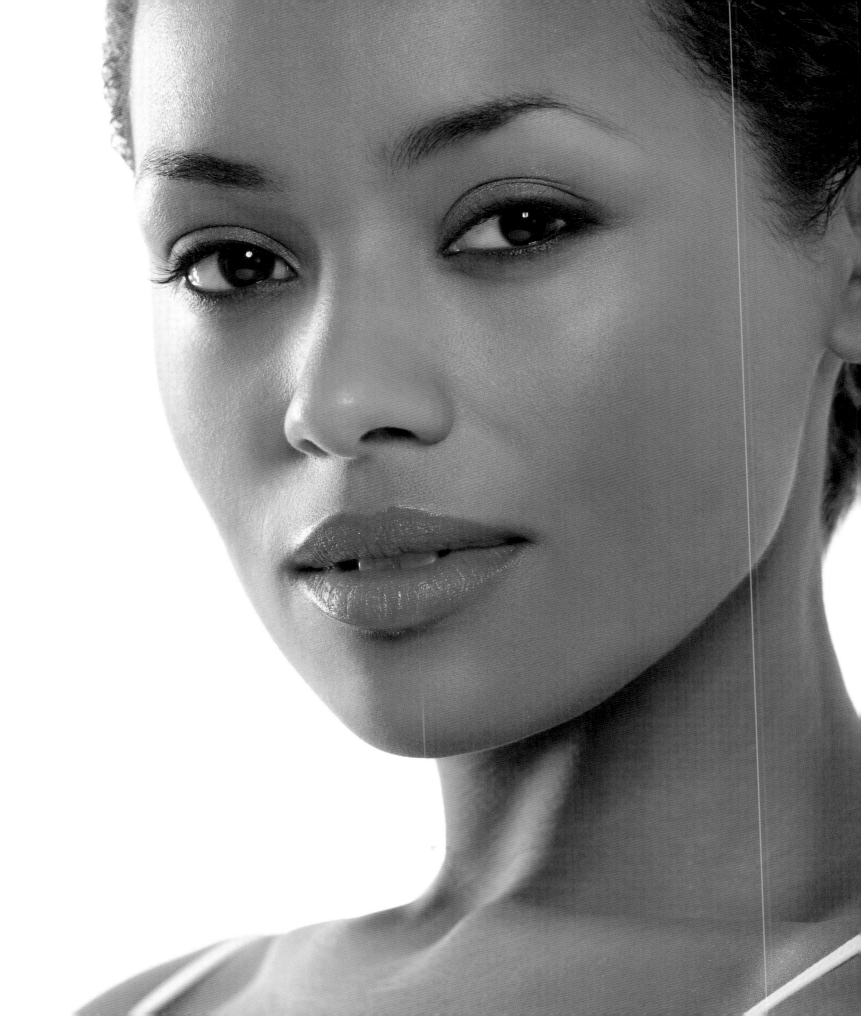

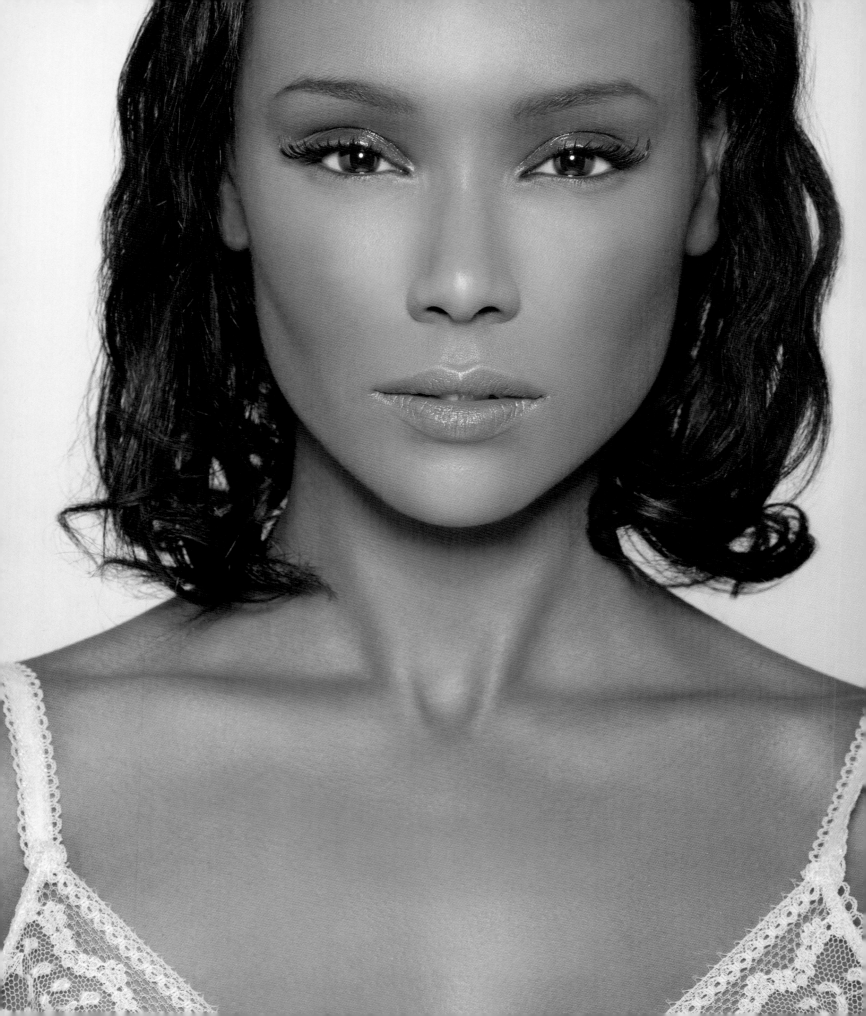

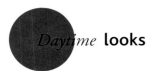

daytime glamour

KEY CONSIDERATIONS

» This look is for a special occasion, so make it different from your everyday or work make-up.

» You need to look natural in daylight, which is less forgiving than low evening lighting.

» A good base is essential to ensure make-up lasts well throughout the day.

For a glamorous lunch party, day at the races, christening or wedding (see also page 167), your make-up should be a little special but still look natural in daylight and not be too 'shouty'. A different approach is called for from when creating a dramatic night-time look, as strong colour, glitter or metallic finishes or heavy eyeliner can seem too much in the bright light of day.

Keep it fresh and pretty, with dewy finishes and soft colours that make your skin glow. I played up the eyes with a fabulous wet-look gloss and false-lash corners. Other features take a back seat, with pale creamy lipstick and a touch of gloss for subtle colour and texture.

Prep your face and eyelids well, as make-up must be long-lasting so that you don't need to take too many products with you, and you can relax without having to carry out constant touch-ups.

TOP TIP

For successful glossy eyes you need big eyelids that are not hooded, otherwise a glossy finish can feel sticky and may crease.

VARIATIONS

» Instead of using gloss on the eyes, cover the eyelid with a neutral eyeshadow to absorb any oil and then apply a wash of shimmering colour – try frosty white or ivory, icy lilac or turquoise.

» Don't use any eyeliner with this look, but curl the lashes and apply a lash tint.

'Don't forget the SPF if you are going to be out in the sun.'

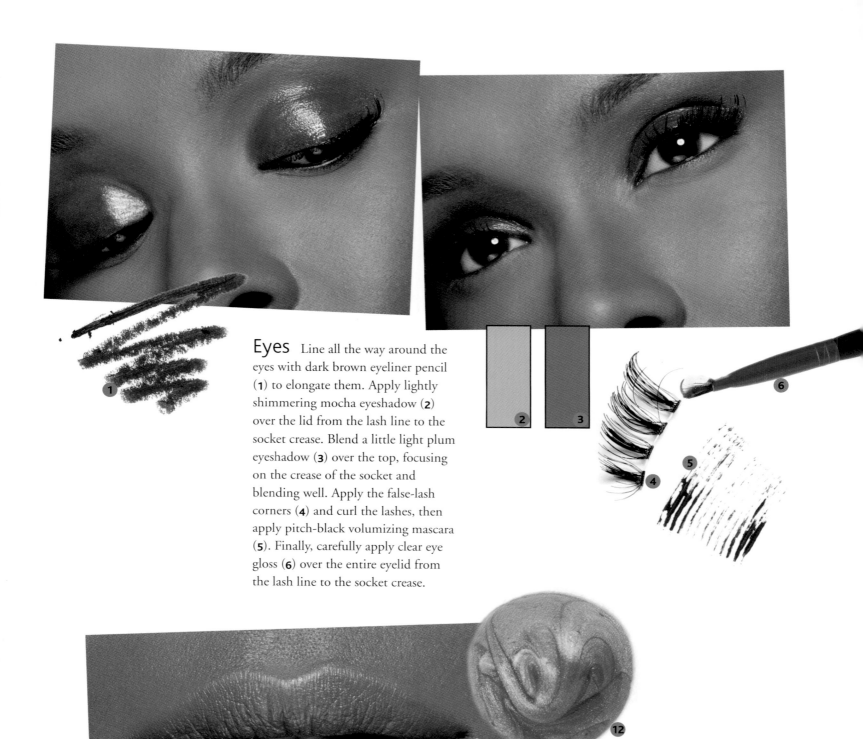

Eyes Line all the way around the eyes with dark brown eyeliner pencil (**1**) to elongate them. Apply lightly shimmering mocha eyeshadow (**2**) over the lid from the lash line to the socket crease. Blend a little light plum eyeshadow (**3**) over the top, focusing on the crease of the socket and blending well. Apply the false-lash corners (**4**) and curl the lashes, then apply pitch-black volumizing mascara (**5**). Finally, carefully apply clear eye gloss (**6**) over the entire eyelid from the lash line to the socket crease.

Lips Apply a touch of foundation around and over the lip line to neutralize their natural colour. Then apply silky pinky-beige lipgloss (**12**) for a lightly shimmering nude finish.

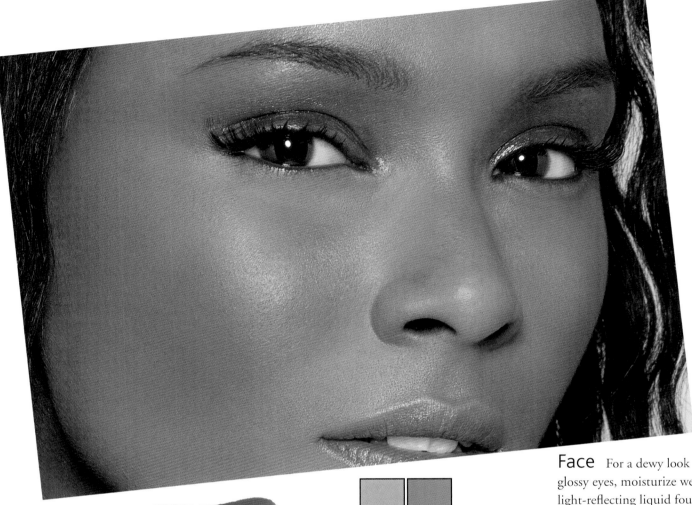

Face For a dewy look that complements glossy eyes, moisturize well and then apply light-reflecting liquid foundation (**7**), with added radiance crème if your skin looks dull. Blend well and apply concealer (**8**) where needed to correct uneven skin tone or blemishes. Take time applying your base to ensure a long-lasting finish. Add fresh pink colour to the apples of the cheeks using crème blush (**9**), softening the edges so that it fades into the skin. Contour the hollow beneath the cheekbones by blending in a little crème bronzer (**10**). Set with a dusting of brightening powder (**11**).

LAST THROUGH LUNCH

Pay lots of attention to your skin. The better moisturized it is, the less likely foundation is to clog or flake.

Try using a primer under your foundation – it will sink into the skin and provide a base that foundation sticks to far better than bare skin. Some primers have radiance products for extra glow.

Spend time applying your foundation, really pushing it into the skin. Add touches of highlighter to cheekbones, browbone and collarbone, and a little sculpting bronzer in the hollows of your temples.

Lip colour that won't rub off when you eat and drink is a good idea. Try a rosy stain for lips and cheeks – apply the stain in a small circle on the apple of your cheek and blend well. Dab onto your lips and add a touch of shimmering gloss.

boardroom beauty

KEY CONSIDERATIONS

» For a work environment, make-up should be natural and subtle in an understated neutral palette.

» The idea is to project a slick, professional image that doesn't stifle your personality.

» Make-up needs to be quick to apply in the morning rush, long-lasting so that you don't need to worry about it during the day, and easy to touch up on the go.

At work you need to be taken seriously, but there's no reason not to enhance your best features and look as good as you can. Knowing that you look your best will boost your confidence and help you to perform better.

The working week is not the time to be experimental with your make-up – stick to neutrals for eyes and lips and save more adventurous looks for weekends and nights out. The most important thing is to appear slick and well groomed at all times, however pressured and stressed you may be feeling on the inside. Keeping your hair and nails conditioned and tidy makes a good impression, while neat defined brows will give your face a strong frame, which suggests an air of authority.

TOP TIPS

» To combat the drying effects of central heating and air conditioning, keep a mineral water spray by your desk to spritz your face, or use a light gel moisturizer that hydrates without disturbing make-up.

» Touch up any redness around tired eyes with a concealer or neutralizing eye base, and draw along the inner rim of the eyes with a pinky-beige eye pencil for a brightening effect.

'Power brows give strength and definition to the face – intensity around the eyes means business.'

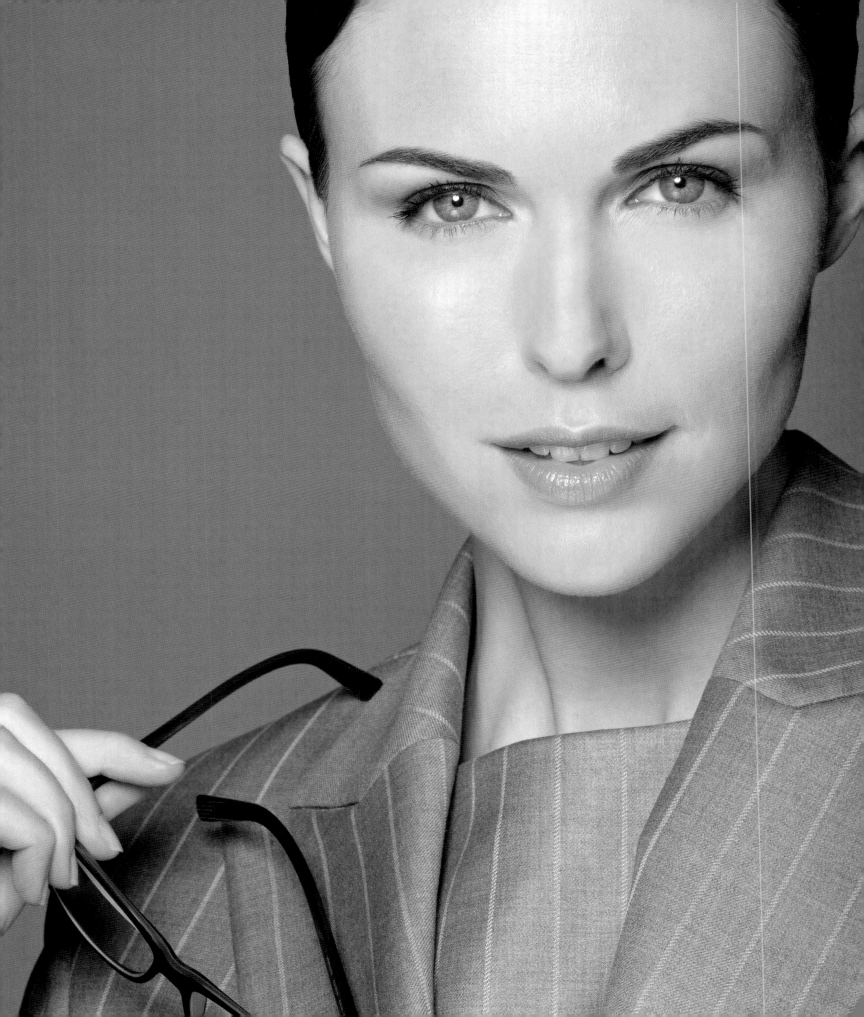

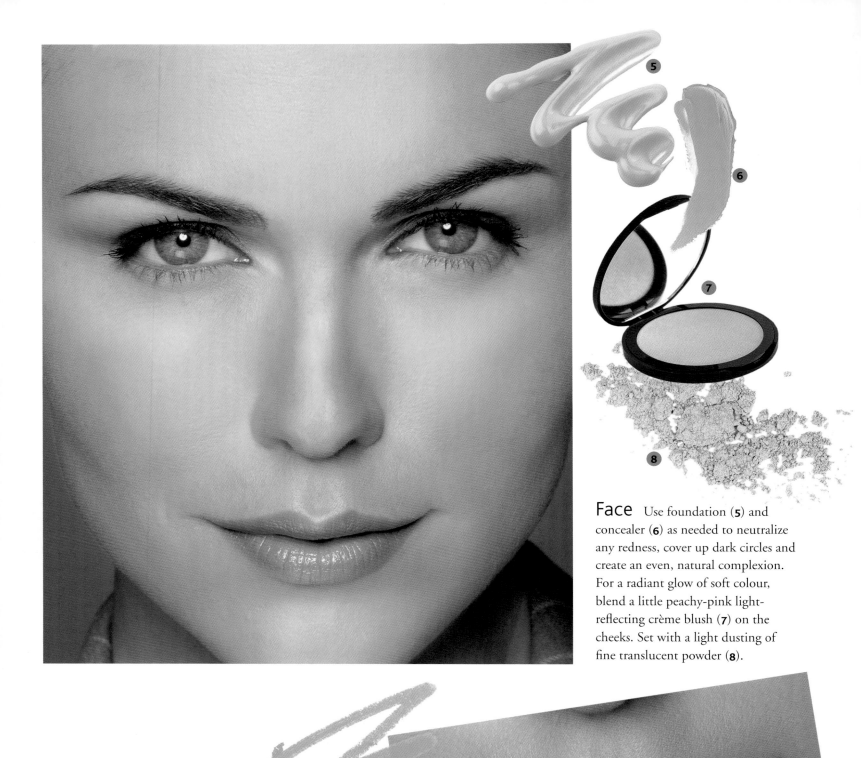

Face Use foundation (**5**) and concealer (**6**) as needed to neutralize any redness, cover up dark circles and create an even, natural complexion. For a radiant glow of soft colour, blend a little peachy-pink light-reflecting crème blush (**7**) on the cheeks. Set with a light dusting of fine translucent powder (**8**).

Lips Outline the lips with a neutral pinky-beige lip pencil (**9**), then fill in the shape – use a brush if necessary to work the pencil into the creases of the lips. Apply petal-pink lipgloss (**10**) and blend over the lips with a brush.

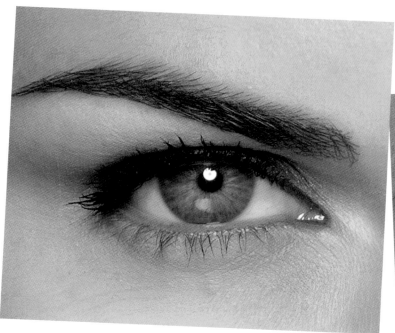

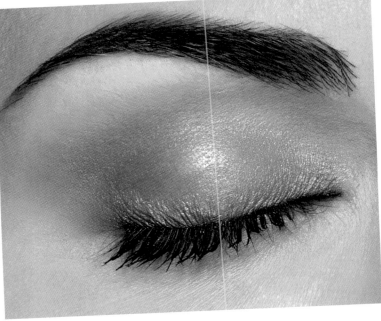

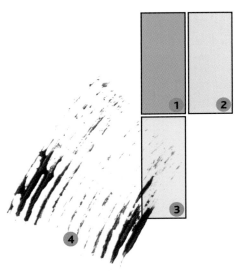

Eyes

Spend time perfecting your brows. Pluck stray hairs and define the shape with a brow pencil and powder, darkening and strengthening them to frame your face. Apply a wash of soft taupe eyeshadow (**1**) over the whole lid area, building up the colour in the crease of the socket at the outer corner of the eye. Blend a pale mushroom shade (**2**) along the lash line and at the inner corner, and brush a little cream highlighter (**3**) over the browbone. Define the lashes with long-lasting lengthening black mascara (**4**).

Girls who wear glasses

» A common mistake is to think that because eyes are behind a barrier, they need to be more dramatically made up, but it's not drama but definition that will help the eyes to stand out.

» Groom your brows to subtly follow the shape of your glasses. Natural brows work best with a straight frame; thin upward-slanting brows with cat's-eye glasses; and the classic arch complements rounded or oval glasses.

» After applying a neutral base, add a darker colour at the lash line and blend up. Blocks of colour work better than subtle gradation. Neutral colours are more flattering with glasses.

» Spend time getting your eyeliner precise at the lash line. On the lower lash line, don't draw on the inner rim as this makes the eye look smaller.

» Shift focus away from the eyes — strong lips look very chic with glasses.

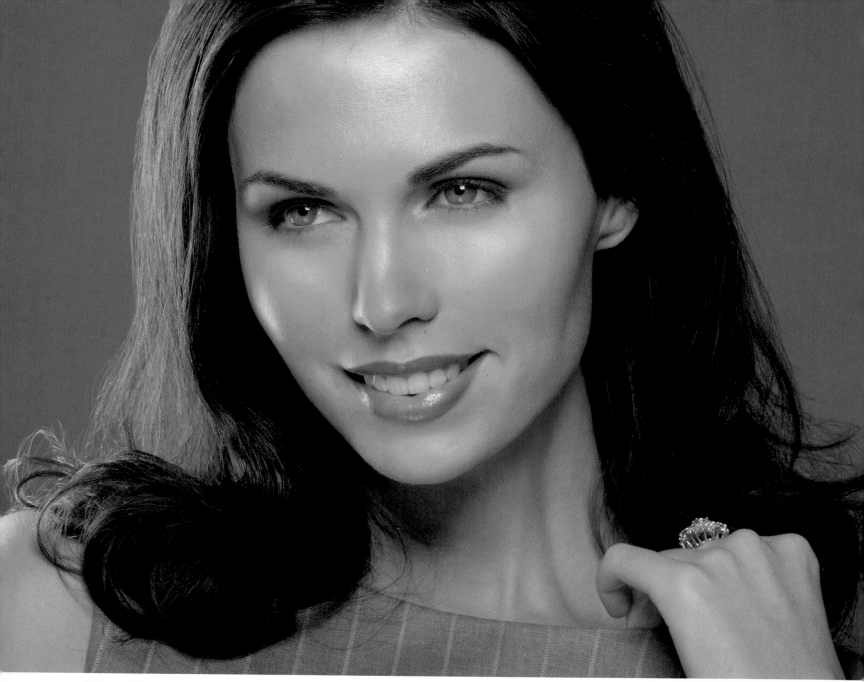

CORPORATE TO COCKTAILS

You need to retain a professional air at a business function or when entertaining clients, but in the evening you can afford to add a little more colour to your look and play up your femininity. In an ideal world, you'll cleanse and reapply foundation (see box opposite), but if you're caught out unexpectedly or pressed for time, you can cut corners. A darker glossy lipstick and more definition around the eyes may be all that's needed to take you from the boardroom to the bar.

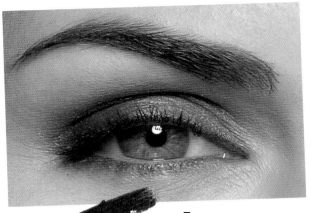

Eyes
Deepen the colour of your eye make-up using a chunky shimmery brown eye crayon (**1**). Draw along the upper lash line and blend with a brush or your finger. Intensify colour in the socket crease, focusing on the outer corners.

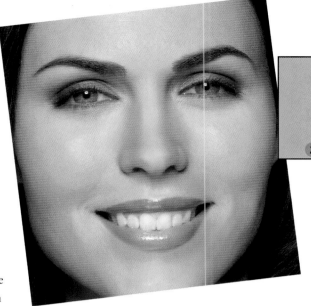

Face
If your base has lasted well, just touch up with concealer as needed. If your skin is looking dull, cleanse with wipes and reapply moisturizer, foundation and concealer. Intensify the colour on your cheeks with fresh pink crème blush (**2**).

EMERGENCY TRANSFORMATION KIT

With these three products you'll always be able to give a neutral daytime look evening glamour.

» Cheek/lip stain – to add an instant flush of colour to cheeks and lips.

» Clear lipgloss – to give lips a glamorous shine and a fuller pout.

» Shimmery brown eye crayon – to define the eyes and build up colour intensity.

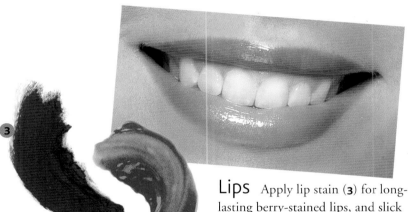

Lips
Apply lip stain (**3**) for long-lasting berry-stained lips, and slick on a coat of pink gloss for a touch of glamour (**4**).

TOP TIPS – FROM DESK TO DINNER

Face
However much of a hurry you're in, spend time on your face – rough or dull skin will ruin any look.

» If foundation looks clogged or dirty, wash your face or cleanse with a wipe.

» Moisturize and pat in foundation until your face looks dewy and fresh. Focus on the front of your cheeks and under the eyes.

» A touch of highlighter on the cheekbones, browbones, bridge of your nose and Cupid's bow will bring light to your face.

Eyes
Change either lips or eyes, not both. If you choose eyes, use a nude gloss on the lips.

» Just add extra eyeliner in a dark colour and smudge it up onto the lid.

» Creamy pencils or shimmering powder eyeshadows apply easily over existing eyeshadow and can be layered for an intense look or smudged for a softer wash of colour.

» For drama, contrast turquoise eyeshadow with black or gold eyeliner. For elegance, pair gold eyeshadow with brown eyeliner.

» Add a touch of highlighter under the browbones and recurl the lashes.

Lips
If you're focusing on lips, keep eyes neutral – just pat translucent powder over the lids to blend out any creases and remove smudges under the eyes with a cotton bud.

» Apply hydrating balm to smooth the lips.

» Outline the lips with a coloured liner, then smudge it into the lips.

» Dab on a creamy lipstick with your fingers to be sure it really sinks in.

» Add a dot of shimmery gloss on the centre of the lower lip.

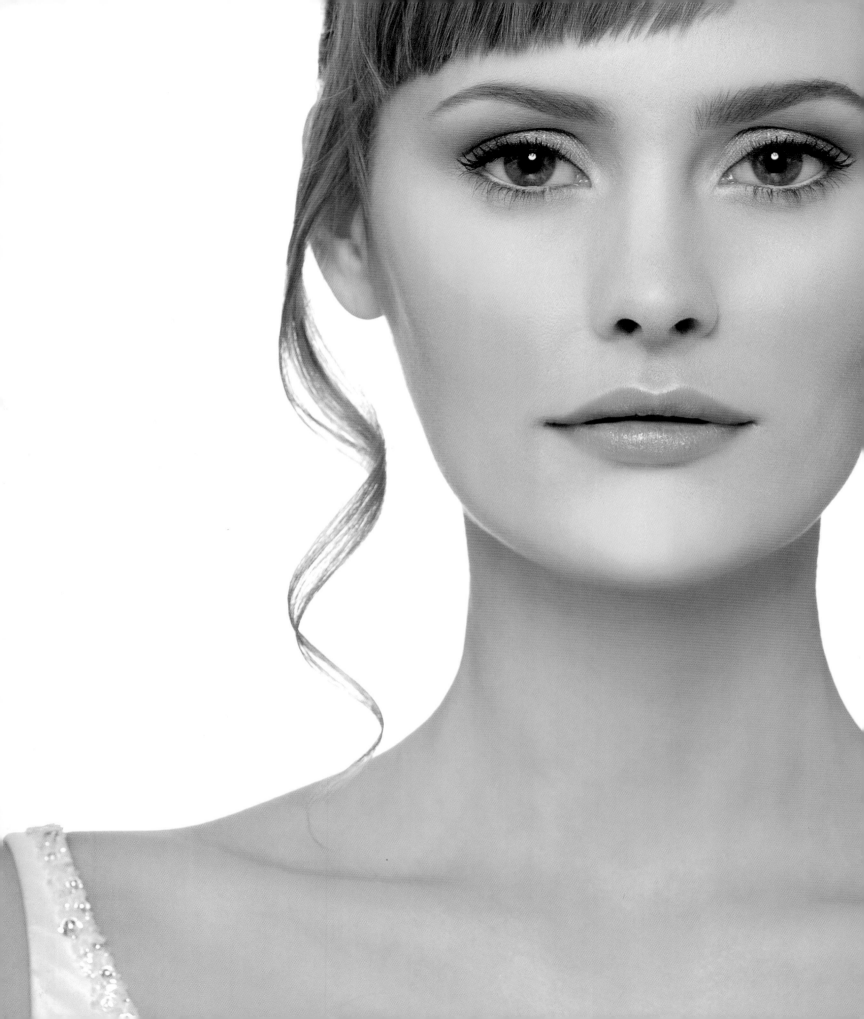

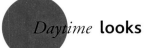

Daytime **looks**

blushing bride

KEY CONSIDERATIONS

» For your wedding more than any other occasion, you want to look stunning but still natural and like yourself.

» Make-up needs to look good in daylight, artificial light and flash photography.

» Formulations should be long-lasting to prevent smudges, so consider water-resistant products if tears are likely.

Every woman wants to be beautiful on her wedding day – radiant in person and stunning in the photos. Make-up should look flattering but natural – it's essential that you look like you and that photos won't look dated in a few years.

The key to successful long-lasting make-up is to spend time preparing the skin beforehand and then creating a flawless base that doesn't look fake or heavy. When applied wrongly, powder can age you – the wrong shade or formula will make your skin look grey and flat in your photos. Mineral foundation is the exception, as it gives a soft, natural finish, is long-lasting and is kind on the skin. Alternatively, use a liquid or crème foundation and set with a fine dusting of light-reflecting translucent powder.

VARIATION

If you're wearing white and have a cool skin tone, a palette of pearl and soft greys is perfect.

» Use a pale highlighter under the brows with a touch at the inner corners of the eyes to keep them looking bright.

» Use a grey pencil to define the outer corners of the upper lid and blend a little darker shadow on top. Add a touch more glamour with a silver pencil for the evening.

» Curl the lashes and use a lash tint for definition without too much volume.

'The best wedding make-up is subtle and unobtrusive, yet reveals and enhances everything that's most beautiful about your face.'

MAID OF HONOUR'S RESCUE KIT

Touch-up concealer – in case of a sudden spot nightmare

Lipgloss – all the kissing quickly wears it off

Tissues – mop up any tears immediately

Blotting tissues – if you have oily skin, these can remove shine

SPF – don't forget this if it's a summer wedding

TOP TIPS

» Plan your look well in advance – a smart city wedding requires a different approach from a traditional country affair.

» Choose a colour palette that enhances the shade of your dress as well as your skin tone.

Eyes

A neutral palette works with any skin tone and is the most straightforward option for beautiful foolproof wedding make-up. First pat a little concealer or eye base over the eyelids to neutralize any redness. Draw a fine line of dark brown eye pencil (**1**) around the eyes, keeping to the roots of the lashes. Draw along the inner rim of the eyes with a flesh-toned eyeliner pencil (**2**) for a brightening effect. Apply a wash of cream eyeshadow (**3**) over the entire eyelid up to the browbone. Add a touch of darker mocha eyeshadow (**4**) at the outer corner of the eye, blending it well into the socket crease. Blend a little shimmering beige eyeshadow (**5**) over the lower part of the lid.

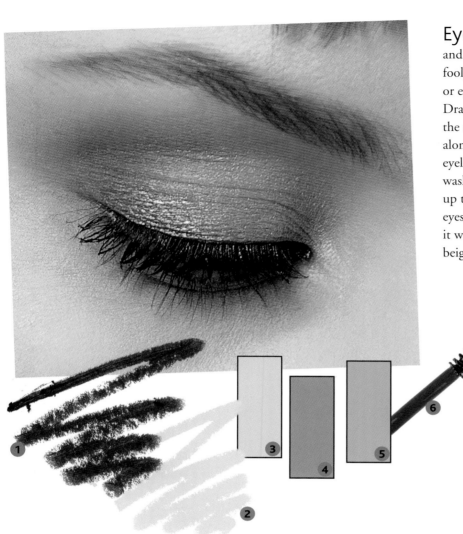

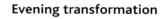

Evening transformation

» To turn up the volume, use a metallic gunmetal eyeliner to darken the eyes.

» Brush a touch of shimmering or glittery powder eyeshadow over the lids.

» Add a hint of shimmering highlighter powder on the cheekbones and under the browbones.

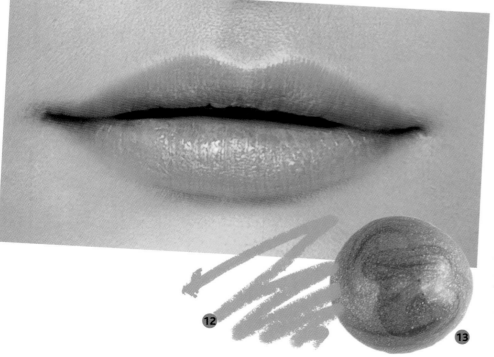

Lips

Outline the lips with a neutral pinky-beige pencil (**12**) and fill in the whole lip area. Then use a sheer lipstick or non-sticky soft rose lipgloss (**13**).

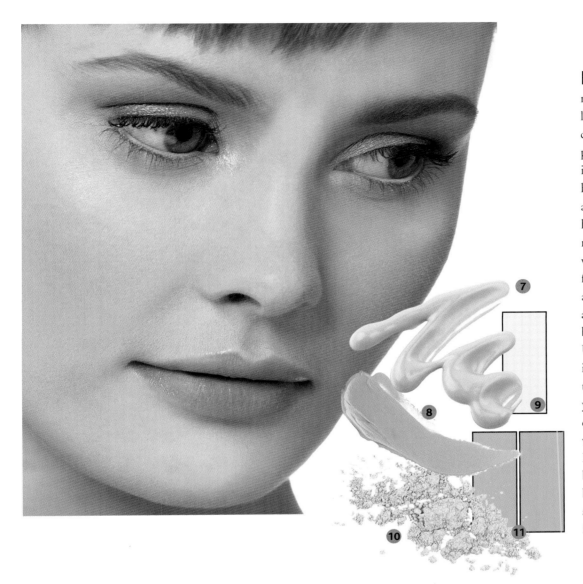

Face For a dewy finish, moisturize thoroughly and let the moisturizer sink in completely before applying primer and foundation. Primer is so important – it helps to hold make-up in place all day and prevents shine. I used a light liquid foundation (**7**), but mineral powder foundation also works well. Don't use too much foundation – just apply it to areas that need it. Neutralize any redness, dark circles or blemishes with concealer (**8**). Use a touch of pinky-cream illuminating crème to highlight the top of the cheekbones (**9**). If you've used liquid foundation, dust the central cross of the face with translucent powder (**10**). For a natural flush, apply a blend of soft peach and sandy-beige powder blush (**11**) to the apples of the cheeks and blend it along the cheekbones.

WEDDING GUEST MAKE-UP

Your make-up needs to look good indoors and out, day and night, and last through tears and dancing. You want to look great in the photos, but remember, this is the bride's day, not yours.

A classic error is to wear a strappy dress, and then use bronzer on the face, so it looks as if a brown face is floating on a white neck and chest. To avoid this, use shimmering body lotion on exfoliated skin.

Powdery finishes can be ageing in daylight, so create dewy skin with radiance crème and tinted moisturizer. Cover blemishes with concealer and dab illuminating crème on cheekbones.

Apply neutral powder under your eye colour to ensure it won't crease. Fresh and innocent is more appropriate than sexy. Try a pastel wash of colour or smudge coloured eyeliner along the top lid.

Add individual fake lashes at the outer corners of the eyes, then define lashes with a long-lasting tint mascara that won't budge for 24 hours.

Fill in lips with lipliner before applying lipstick, then blot and reapply for a long-lasting finish. All you need take with you is a non-sticky gloss for occasional touch-ups.

'If you're wearing a bright lip colour, remember to air-kiss.'

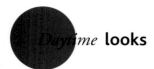

yummy mummy

KEY CONSIDERATIONS

» When you're a mother, the most valuable commodity is time: make-up needs to be super-quick to apply.

» You want to look well-groomed and fabulously natural – the aim is to create a brighter, fresher appearance, as though you've had eight hours' uninterrupted sleep.

» Multitasking formulas containing hydrating, antiageing and skin-brightening ingredients and two-in-one products are lifesavers.

Finding time to apply make-up can seem impossible when you're juggling nappy changes, school runs, work and family. But there are some time-saving skills and products that will help you to achieve beautiful make-up in less time.

This look is not a statement one, but very natural and barely there. Make-up is used to illuminate the skin, brighten and open up the eyes and bring a little healthy colour to the cheeks.

Choose 'skintelligent' light-reflecting formulations to hydrate, firm, brighten and reduce the visibility of fine lines. Colours should be neutral, soft and subtle, enhancing and flattering your complexion. For the most wearable look, textures should be neutral, too – neither too matte nor too dewy, although a light shimmer on the eyes has a brightening effect that will counteract any tiredness.

TOP TIP

For the cheapest, fastest facial, bathe your face in warm water and then cold – this stimulates the circulation and makes your skin glow.

DAY-TO-NIGHT TRANSFORMATION

Touch up your base as necessary and outline your eyes with a dark brown pencil. Smooth out any creases on your eyeshadow with a cotton bud, then blend a little shimmer powder over the top and apply highlighter to the browbone. Curl your lashes and add another coat of mascara. Apply creamy lipstick in a deeper colour than your daytime gloss.

'A combination of clever techniques, "skintelligent" ingredients and multipurpose products makes it easy for mums on the go to perfect a time-efficient day look.'

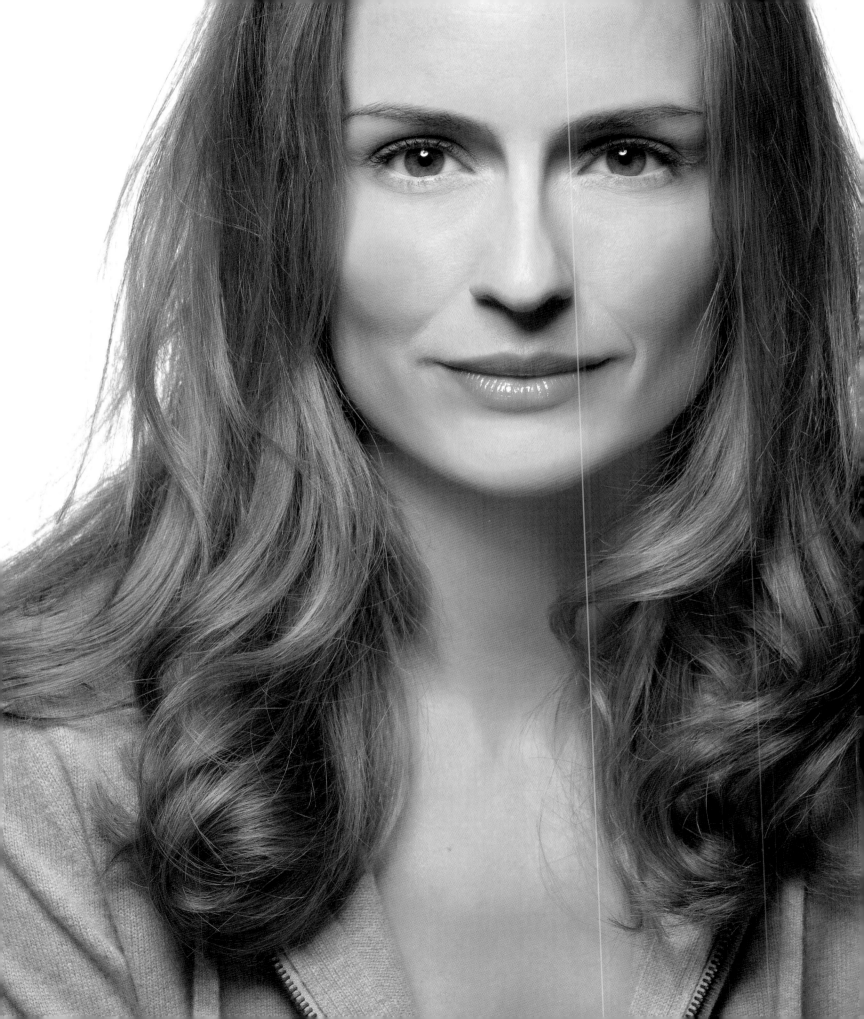

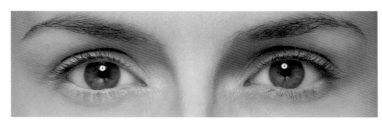

Eyes

Lack of sleep can make eyes look red and tired, so a soothing crème base to neutralize red lids and a flesh-toned eyeliner pencil to brighten the eyes are invaluable (see right). Apply a liquid eyeshadow in a soft pale brown (**1**) over the lid and up to the socket crease. Choose a cooling silky formula that will glide on easily and contains firming antiageing ingredients. Curl the lashes and apply a coat of non-smudging lengthening brown mascara (**2**).

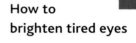

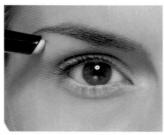

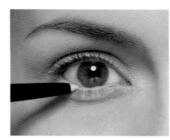

How to brighten tired eyes

Dab a little antiageing flesh-coloured crème around the eyes and over the lids and blend well. This will reduce any redness caused by tiredness and even out skin tone; it also acts as a primer and base for eyeshadow. Next, apply flesh-toned eyeliner along the inner rim of the lower lid, just above the lash line, to open up the eyes.

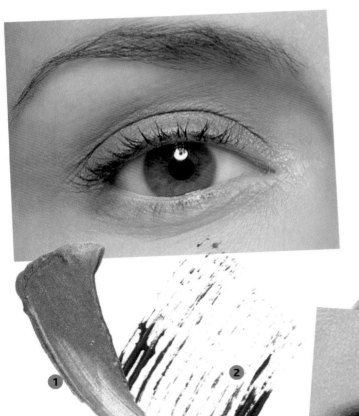

Lips

Apply rosy stain (**7**) to the lips, blending with your finger or pressing your lips together to distribute the colour evenly. This gives natural long-lasting colour. Apply a little pale pink lipgloss (**8**) over the top.

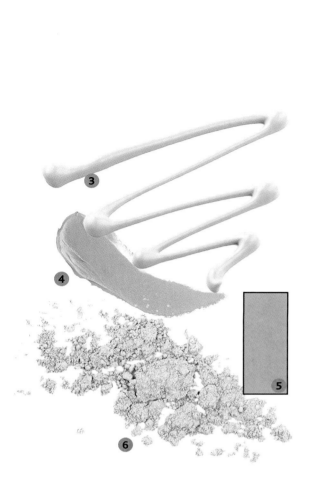

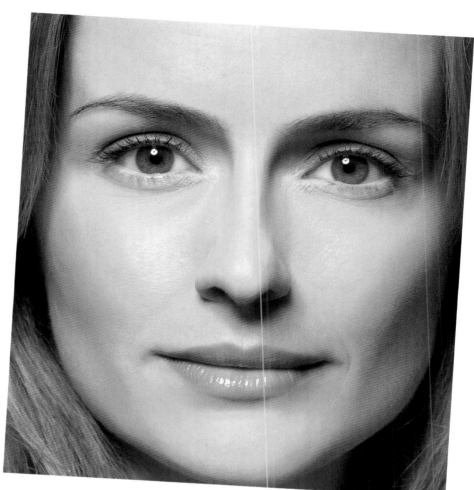

Face

If your complexion is good, use tinted moisturizer (**3**) – a good corner-cutting product for everyday wear. If you need more coverage, after moisturizing, apply a hydrating, light-reflecting foundation wherever you need it to even out skin tone and brighten up tired-looking skin. Choose a formulation rich in skincare ingredients to make up for a time-poor beauty regime. Apply concealer (**4**) as needed and blend well to cover dark circles under the eyes. For a natural flush, blend fresh pink crème blush (**5**) onto the apples of the cheeks. To prevent shine, dust the central cross of the face with translucent powder (**6**).

HANDBAG ESSENTIALS

There are times when you rush out fresh-faced and natural, then later wish you had brought a couple of products with you. Here are my multitasking essentials that can transform your look with ease.

CONCEALER
Touches of concealer are often all you need. Mask redness around the nose or chin and cover up dark undereye circles.

JUMBO EYE CRAYONS
These creamy pencils are eyeshadow and eyeliner in one, and you don't need brushes to apply them. Draw a line at the lashes and blend up towards the socket with your finger. You can then either colour a line just above the socket and smudge gently, or increase the intensity of colour at the lash line.

LIP AND CHEEK STAIN
Unlike powder blush, this blends well on bare skin so there's no need to carry translucent powder. Paint a circle on the apple of your cheek and blend with your fingers for a natural flush. It also gives a rosy, bee-stung pout to lips.

DUAL ILLUMINATOR
To take a look from day to night, the crème highlighter can be used on eyelids, under browbones, on cheekbones, on the décolletage and even on the lips. The shimmer dust makes a great eyeshadow and can be used on collarbones and cheekbones to revitalize tired-looking skin.

NIGHT-
TIME

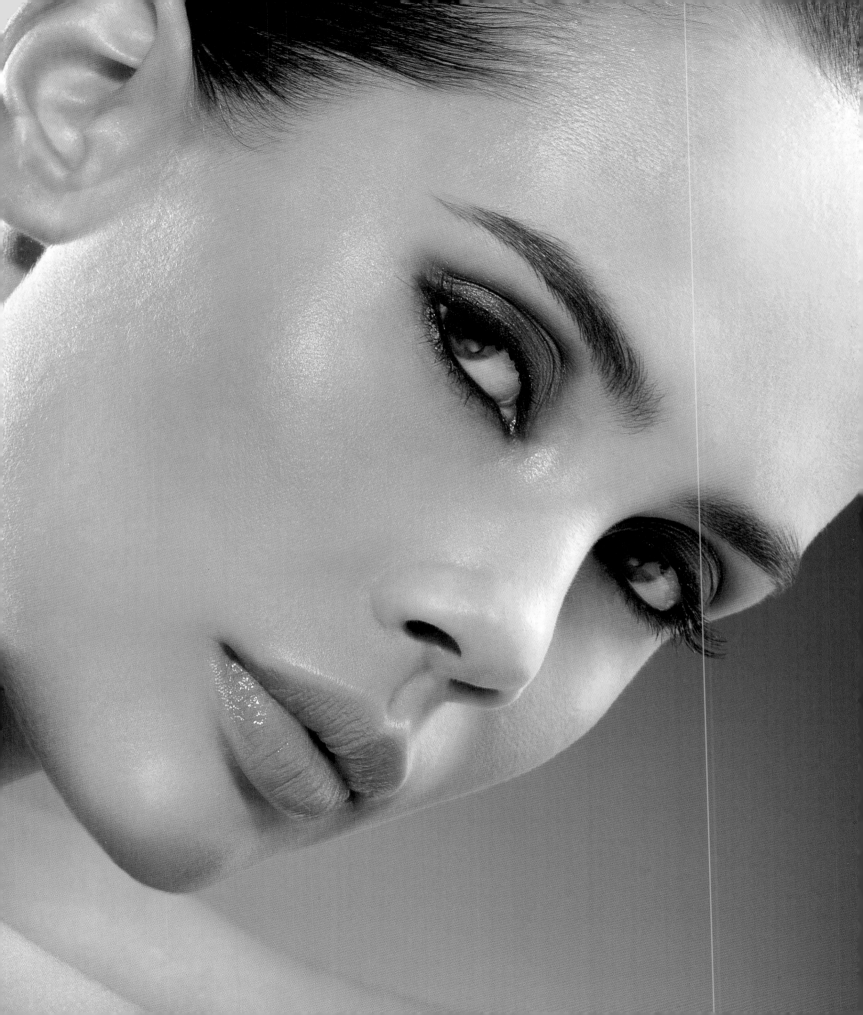

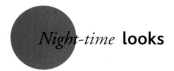

after-dark beauty

This is elegant evening make-up that makes a statement but is very wearable. The emphasis is on glamour, with colours chosen to flatter skin tone. At night dark colours – from neutral greys to rich jewel tones – smoulder and look sultry, while glitter and metallic finishes that seem garish during the day glimmer alluringly and add drama. Play around with texture, combining different finishes on the eyes, lips and face – shimmer, matte and gloss finishes for eyes or lips all work well with a matte, semi-matte or dewy complexion.

porcelain

The classic smoky eye is particularly flattering on cool pink-based skin tones, as shades of steely grey look fabulous against pale porcelain skin. The sculpted matte base, metallic crème eyeshadow and slightly glossy lips create an interesting play on textures.

Eyes Ensure the brows are groomed and defined. Outline the eyes with a pitch-black eye pencil (**1**), working the tip between the roots of the lashes to make them look thicker. Apply a wash of cloudy-grey powder shadow (**2**) up to the browbone. Blend dark grey eyeshadow (**3**) along the lash line, blending it over the pencil eyeliner. Use a synthetic brush to apply gunmetal metallic crème eyeshadow (**4**) above the eyeliner, blending it up to the socket crease. Curl the lashes and apply volumizing black mascara (**5**).

Lips Pat rosy lip stain (**10**) into the lips. When it is dry, brush a little pink lipgloss (**11**) onto the centre of the lower lip and press the lips together to blend.

Face For flawless skin use matte foundation (**6**) and apply concealer (**7**) wherever you need it to cover dark circles or blemishes. Set with fine translucent powder (**8**) for an even velvety finish. Lightly dust the cheeks with soft pink powder blush (**9**) – nothing too strong so the face remains creamy and pale with a touch of colour.

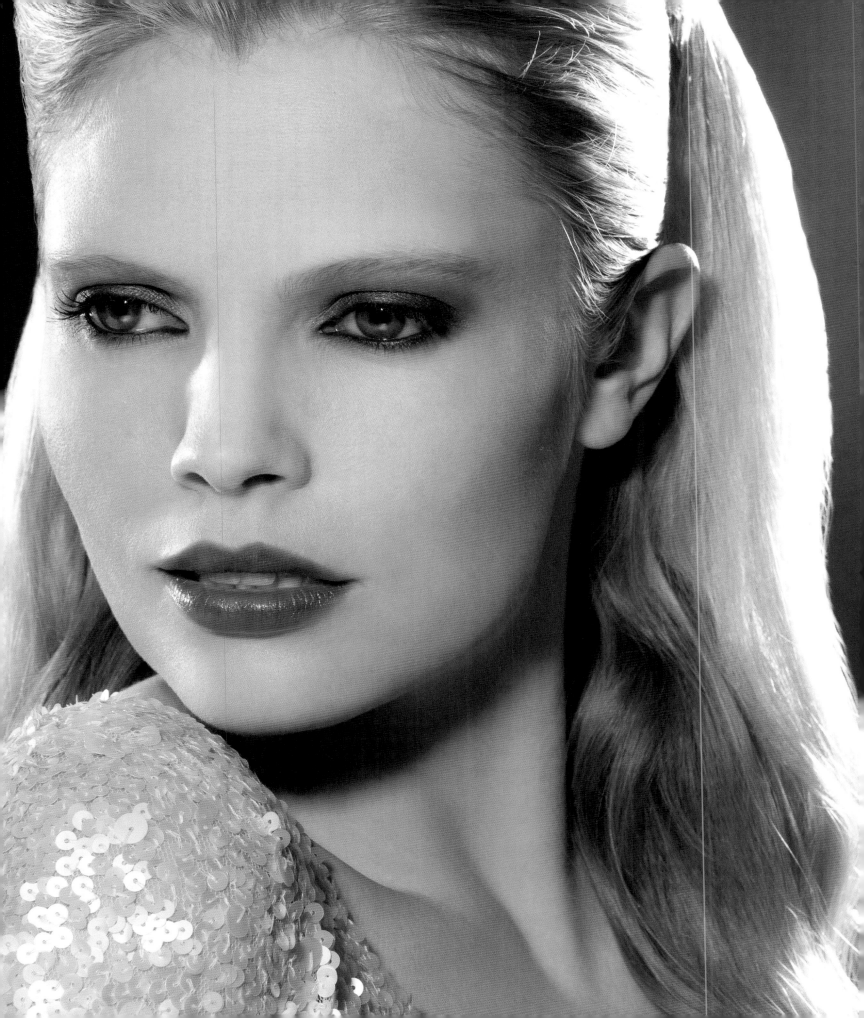

fair

Don't be afraid to use colour on your eyes. Midnight blue and sapphire look stunning if you have blue or hazel eyes, while violet blue with a purple undertone enhances green eyes. Semi-matte skin and glossy lips in understated neutrals keep the focus on the smouldering eyes.

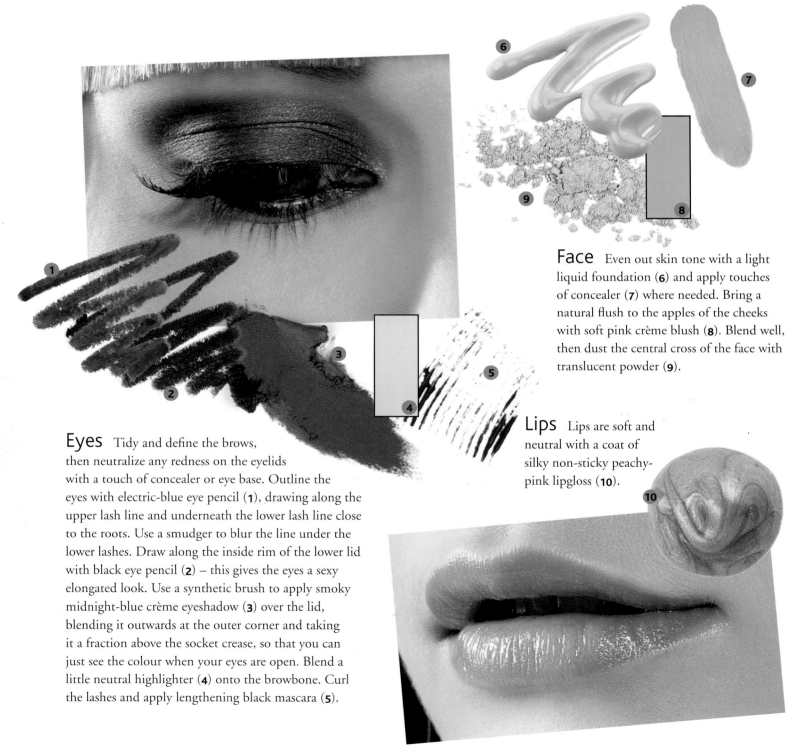

Face
Even out skin tone with a light liquid foundation (**6**) and apply touches of concealer (**7**) where needed. Bring a natural flush to the apples of the cheeks with soft pink crème blush (**8**). Blend well, then dust the central cross of the face with translucent powder (**9**).

Eyes
Tidy and define the brows, then neutralize any redness on the eyelids with a touch of concealer or eye base. Outline the eyes with electric-blue eye pencil (**1**), drawing along the upper lash line and underneath the lower lash line close to the roots. Use a smudger to blur the line under the lower lashes. Draw along the inside rim of the lower lid with black eye pencil (**2**) – this gives the eyes a sexy elongated look. Use a synthetic brush to apply smoky midnight-blue crème eyeshadow (**3**) over the lid, blending it outwards at the outer corner and taking it a fraction above the socket crease, so that you can just see the colour when your eyes are open. Blend a little neutral highlighter (**4**) onto the browbone. Curl the lashes and apply lengthening black mascara (**5**).

Lips
Lips are soft and neutral with a coat of silky non-sticky peachy-pink lipgloss (**10**).

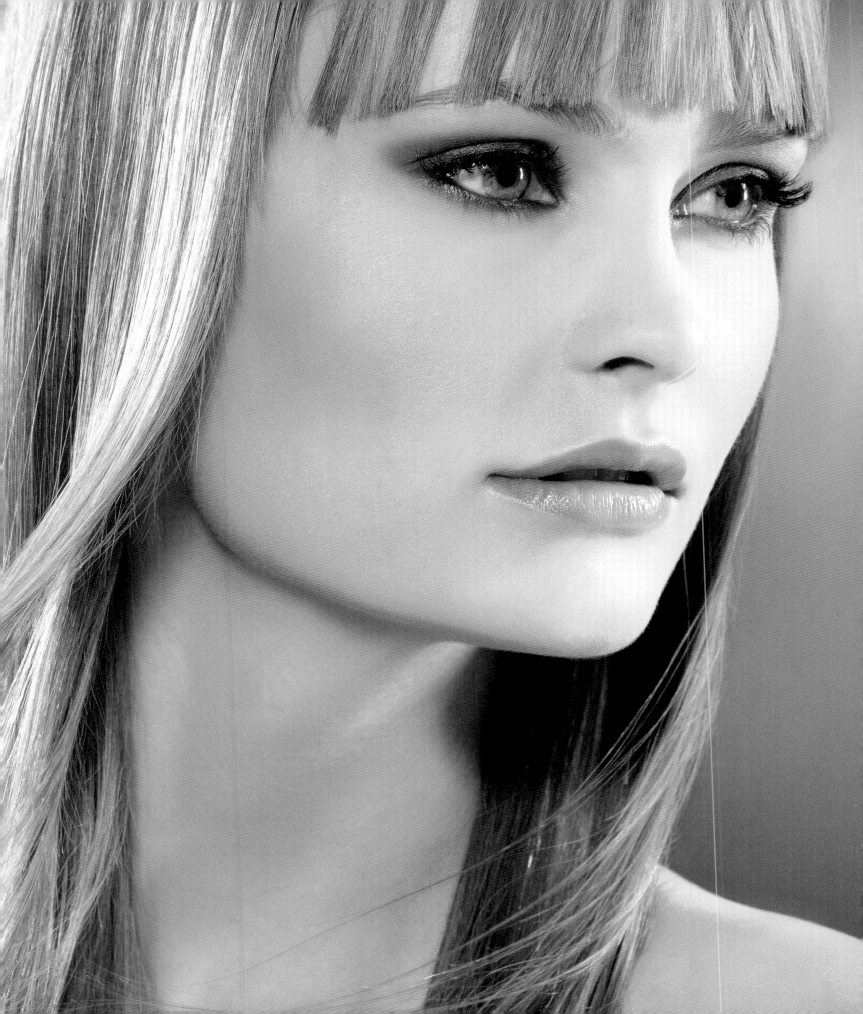

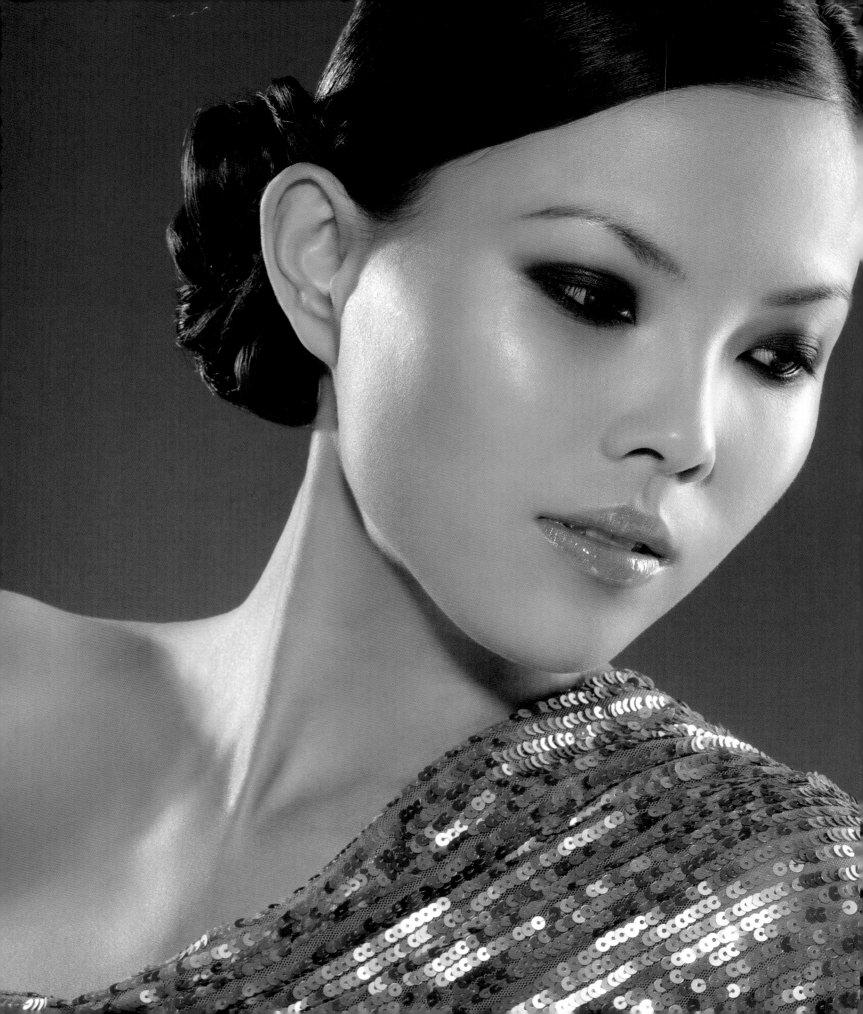

light olive

This is a smoky eye with a twist. Instead of classic shades of grey, mocha and dark bronze complement the warmer yellow-based skin tone and intensify brown eyes. The eyes are elegantly offset by hints of pink on the cheeks and lips.

Eyes Groom and shape the brows, then outline the eye with a mahogany eye pencil (**1**), drawing along the upper lash line and just underneath the roots of the lower lashes. Blur the line under the eye with a smudger for a smoky effect. Draw along the inner rim of the lower lid with a black pencil (**2**) to elongate the eyes. Use a synthetic brush to apply dark purply bronze crème eyeshadow (**3**) over the lid from the lash line to the socket crease, taking the colour just high enough so that it can be seen when your eyes are open. Using a natural brush, blend a little shimmery mocha eyeshadow (**4**) on top. Blend a touch of rose-gold highlighter (**5**) on the browbone. Coat the lashes with lengthening black mascara (**6**).

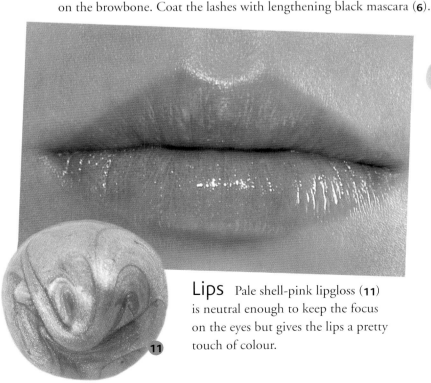

Lips Pale shell-pink lipgloss (**11**) is neutral enough to keep the focus on the eyes but gives the lips a pretty touch of colour.

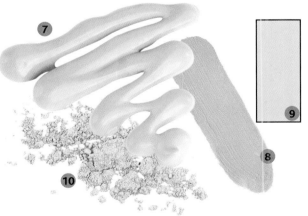

Face Apply light liquid foundation (**7**) to even out skin tone and blend concealer (**8**) where needed to hide any blemishes. Add a touch of soft pink to the apples of the cheeks using crème blush (**9**) and blend a little rose-gold highlighter (**5**) along the top of the cheekbones. Lightly brush the face with translucent powder (**10**).

dark olive

Dark olive skin, which can look sallow, is warmed up with bronzer to give a sunkissed glow. Nude gloss enhances full lips without detracting from stunning metallic green eyes.

Eyes Ensure the brows are groomed, then outline the eyes with a black eyeliner pencil (**1**), working the tip between the roots of the lashes to create extra volume. Use a smudger to soften the line below the lower lashes. Draw along the upper lash line with a black gel eyeliner (**2**). Apply metallic green eyeshadow (**3**) over the lid from the lash line to the socket crease and use a touch of neutral highlighter (**4**) on the browbone. Curl the lashes and coat with volumizing black mascara (**5**).

Face Even out skin tone with a light liquid foundation (**6**) or a mineral foundation if your skin is prone to oiliness. Apply concealer (**7**) where needed to hide any flaws. If you've used liquid foundation, dust lightly with translucent powder (**8**). For a sunkissed glow, sweep bronzing powder (**9**) onto the cheeks and blend well.

Lips Moisturize lips with nude tinted lip balm (**10**), then top with a nude gloss (**11**) to make them look luscious and full.

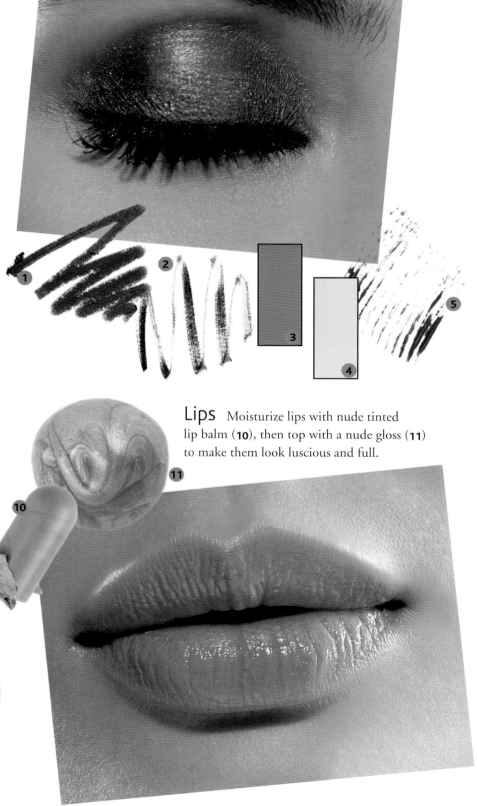

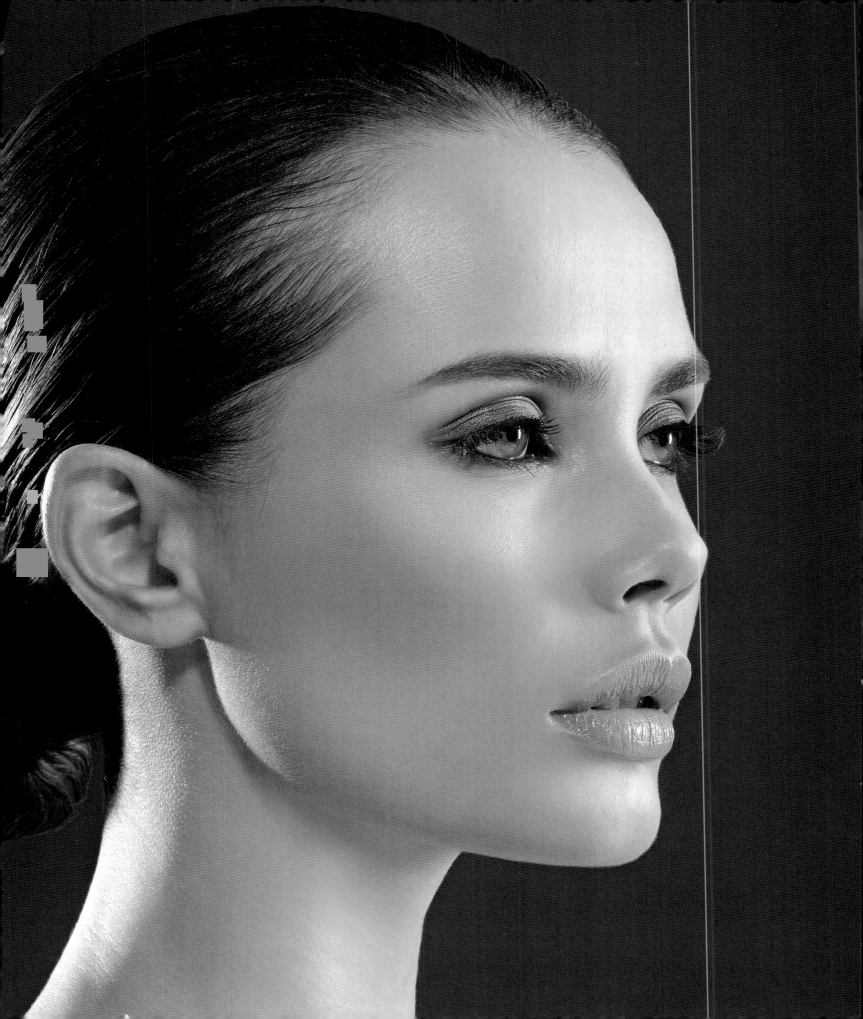

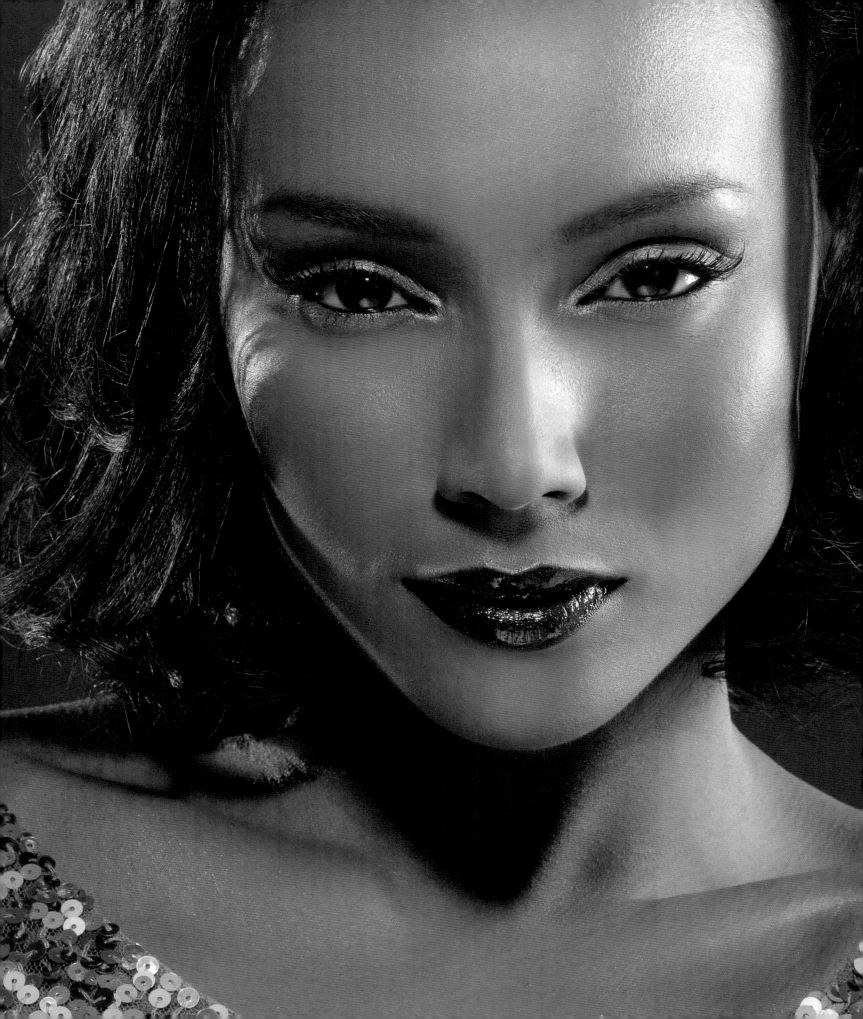

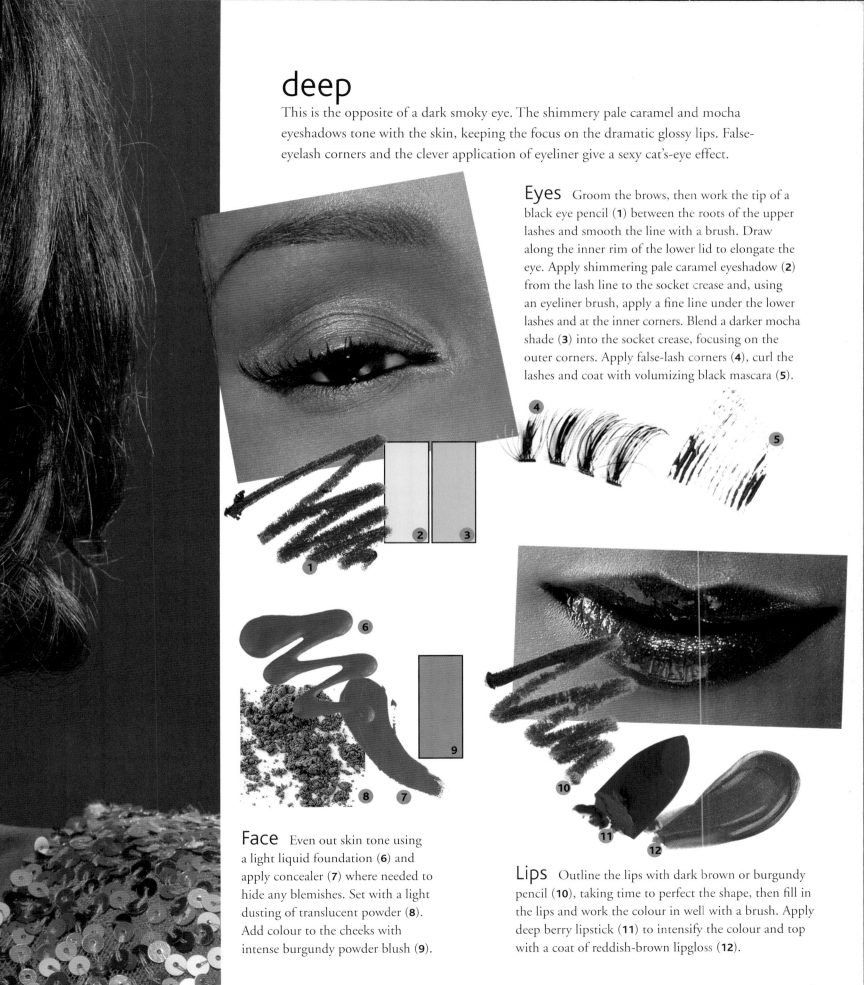

deep

This is the opposite of a dark smoky eye. The shimmery pale caramel and mocha eyeshadows tone with the skin, keeping the focus on the dramatic glossy lips. False-eyelash corners and the clever application of eyeliner give a sexy cat's-eye effect.

Eyes Groom the brows, then work the tip of a black eye pencil (**1**) between the roots of the upper lashes and smooth the line with a brush. Draw along the inner rim of the lower lid to elongate the eye. Apply shimmering pale caramel eyeshadow (**2**) from the lash line to the socket crease and, using an eyeliner brush, apply a fine line under the lower lashes and at the inner corners. Blend a darker mocha shade (**3**) into the socket crease, focusing on the outer corners. Apply false-lash corners (**4**), curl the lashes and coat with volumizing black mascara (**5**).

Face Even out skin tone using a light liquid foundation (**6**) and apply concealer (**7**) where needed to hide any blemishes. Set with a light dusting of translucent powder (**8**). Add colour to the cheeks with intense burgundy powder blush (**9**).

Lips Outline the lips with dark brown or burgundy pencil (**10**), taking time to perfect the shape, then fill in the lips and work the colour in well with a brush. Apply deep berry lipstick (**11**) to intensify the colour and top with a coat of reddish-brown lipgloss (**12**).

foxy and fabulous

KEY CONSIDERATIONS

» This look is traditionally achieved with liquid eyeliner, but gel liner is easier to apply and gives a similar finish. Pencil eyeliner creates a softer line with blurred edges.

» The eyeliner is what makes the statement, so choose subtle eyeshadows that blend with your skin tone.

» Understated lipstick gives the look a soft, contemporary feel.

VARIATION

» For extra va-va-voom, go for glossy berry-red lips.

The classic 1950s flick was made famous by glamorous Hollywood sirens such as Marilyn Monroe, and conjures up images of smoky bars, jazz bands and martinis. It's a timeless sexy look that's not for shrinking violets.

For a modern feel, the face is peaches-and-cream pale with a velvety matte finish, and lips are pretty and light in glossy fresh pink. The dramatic eyeliner creates the impact, so the eyeshadow is kept pale and neutral with just a little depth of colour in the socket crease for definition. False-eyelash corners and lashings of mascara complete the seductive heavy-lidded look.

'This is a go-anywhere look that works as well with jeans and wedges as it does with a cocktail dress and killer heels.'

TOP TIPS

» Rest your elbow on a table as you draw the flick to help steady your hand.

» Use a cotton bud dipped in eye make-up remover to wipe away mistakes.

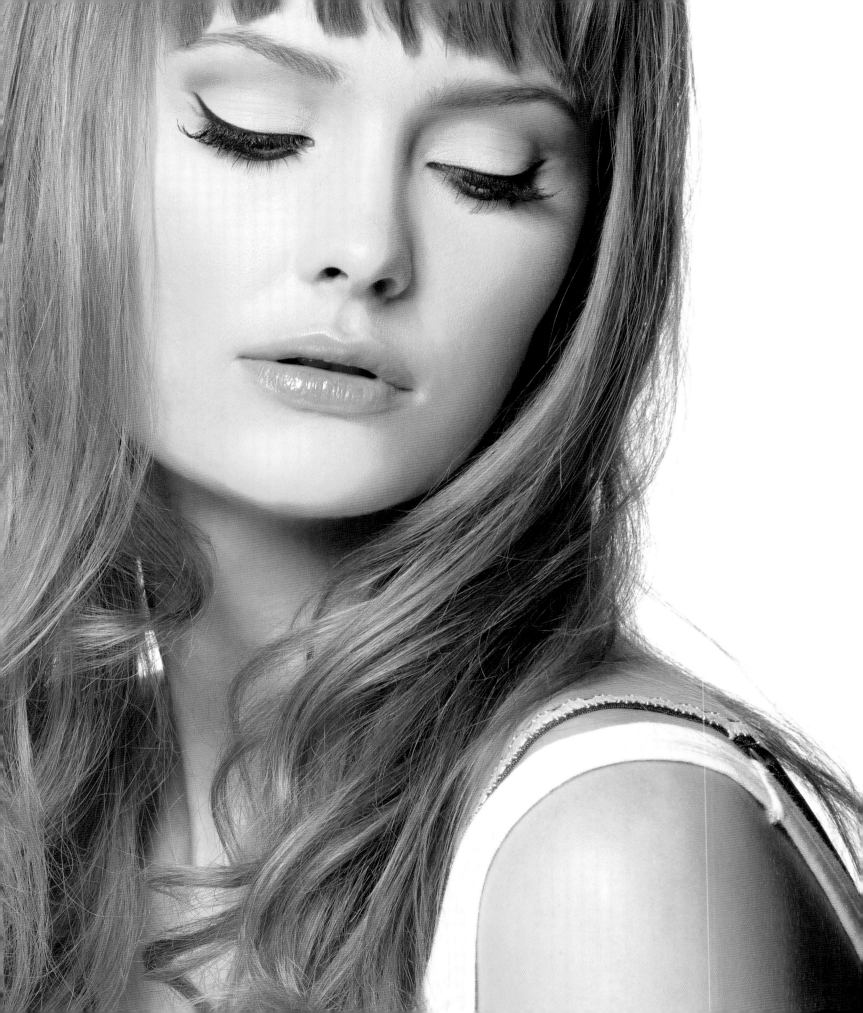

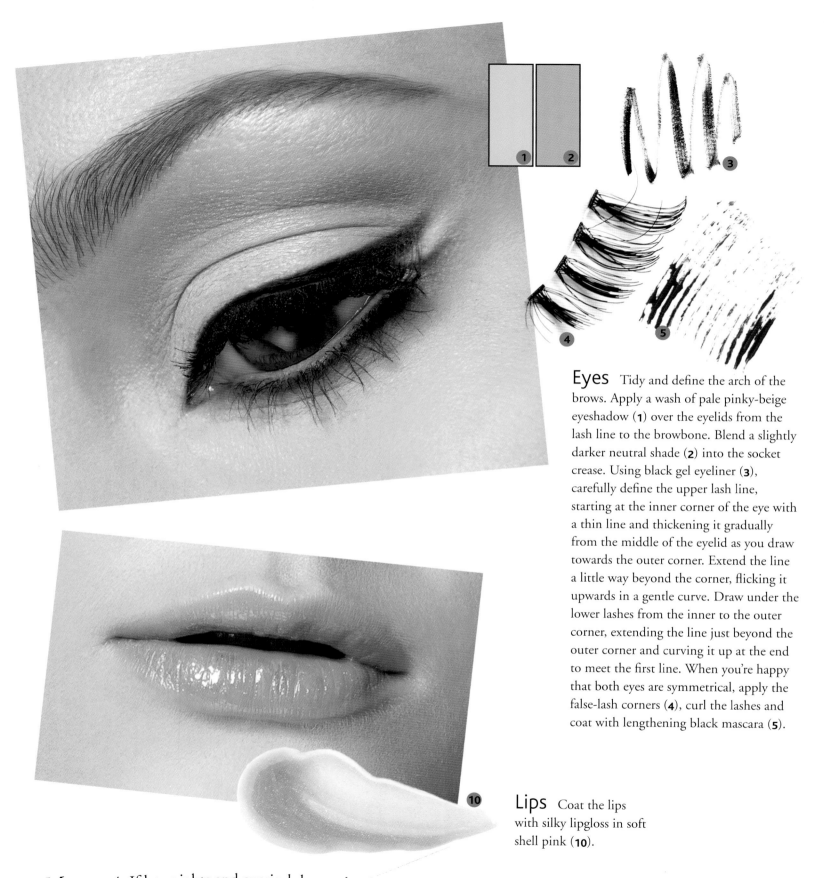

Eyes Tidy and define the arch of the brows. Apply a wash of pale pinky-beige eyeshadow (**1**) over the eyelids from the lash line to the browbone. Blend a slightly darker neutral shade (**2**) into the socket crease. Using black gel eyeliner (**3**), carefully define the upper lash line, starting at the inner corner of the eye with a thin line and thickening it gradually from the middle of the eyelid as you draw towards the outer corner. Extend the line a little way beyond the corner, flicking it upwards in a gentle curve. Draw under the lower lashes from the inner to the outer corner, extending the line just beyond the outer corner and curving it up at the end to meet the first line. When you're happy that both eyes are symmetrical, apply the false-lash corners (**4**), curl the lashes and coat with lengthening black mascara (**5**).

Lips Coat the lips with silky lipgloss in soft shell pink (**10**).

My secret If late nights and overindulgence lead to a breakout, apply a little neat tea tree oil with a cotton bud. Then dab a touch of concealer on top and blend only at the edges, never on the spot itself.

MORNING-AFTER SKIN Here's my rescue plan for dull, partied-out skin.

CLEANSE However late you get home, remove your make-up – it's best to use a cleanser, but at the very least take off eye make-up with wipes – and moisturize. Drink a large glass of water with lemon – replenishing moisture will do more good than anything you can do with make-up.

EXFOLIATE Gently exfoliate away dead skin cells, which can make skin look lifeless. Ingredients to look for are: green tea and aloe to calm, lemon oil for an illuminating effect, and essential oils to soften.

DE-PUFF Jump-start your circulation by applying alternate hot and cold compresses.

MOISTURIZE Use a hydrating face mask containing cucumber or antioxidants to purify and revitalize. Use serum under your moisturizer – if your skin is dry, use a rehydrating serum; if it looks dull, choose one to brighten the skin. Rehydrate the eye area with a light gel and use a rich balm on your lips.

MAKE-UP Have a break from 'full' make-up. Use tinted moisturizer or radiance crème to make skin glow, and set with a little translucent powder for a velvety finish. Dab radiance crème on the cheekbones, nose, eyelids and browbones – a subtle sheen is a lifesaver for tired skin. Bronzer can add a touch of sun, but be careful not to overdo it – sheer crème will look more natural than powder. Or, for a healthy flush, apply rose-pink blush or stain to the apples of your cheeks – this adds brightness to a tired face without being obvious. On your eyes, use a very creamy or liquid illuminating concealer one shade lighter than your skin to brighten and hide shadows, then apply mascara. Moisturize lips with tinted lip balm.

Face

Apply liquid foundation (**6**) to even out the skin tone and blend concealer (**7**) where needed for a flawless finish. Dust the face with translucent powder (**8**) for a velvety finish and apply soft peachy-beige powder blush to the cheeks (**9**).

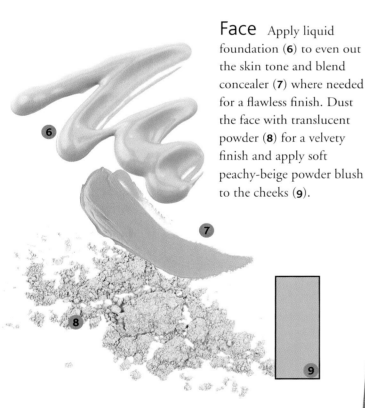

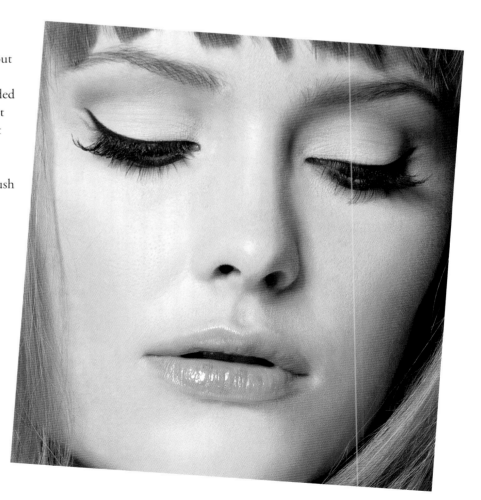

red-carpet glamour

KEY CONSIDERATIONS

» This is sophisticated make-up that spells grown-up glamour and elegance – think Grace Kelly.

» The crucial element is a totally flawless complexion, so allow plenty of time to prepare the skin well and apply foundation to ensure a long-lasting base.

» The striking red lips will draw the eye, so precise application is essential.

VARIATION

» For a subtler red lip, use a sheer lipstick or a lip stain with a touch of gloss.

Here is the ultimate red-carpet look to set off a show-stopping dress and unfeasibly high heels. This timeless make-up can't be beaten for special occasions when you want to look groomed and polished – you'll feel like a million dollars, even without George Clooney on your arm.

A perfect radiant complexion is crucial, so make sure you get this right with plenty of prep, an illuminating primer under foundation, a perfect colour match for your base and the correct formulation for your skin – liquid foundation absorbs well and is less likely to show in creases than a heavier formulation, but if you prefer a mineral foundation, buff it really well to be sure it has absorbed properly.

Eyes should be neutral to keep the look understated and elegant, so choose eyeshadow colours that are close to your natural skin tone.

'Experiment with different shades of red lipstick to find one that suits your colouring.'

TOP TIPS

» Foundation that is too pale or too dark will show up in photographs – if you can't find the perfect match for your skin tone, blend two shades together.

» Work foundation onto your throat and décolletage, too, patting it in thoroughly so that none will come off on your dress.

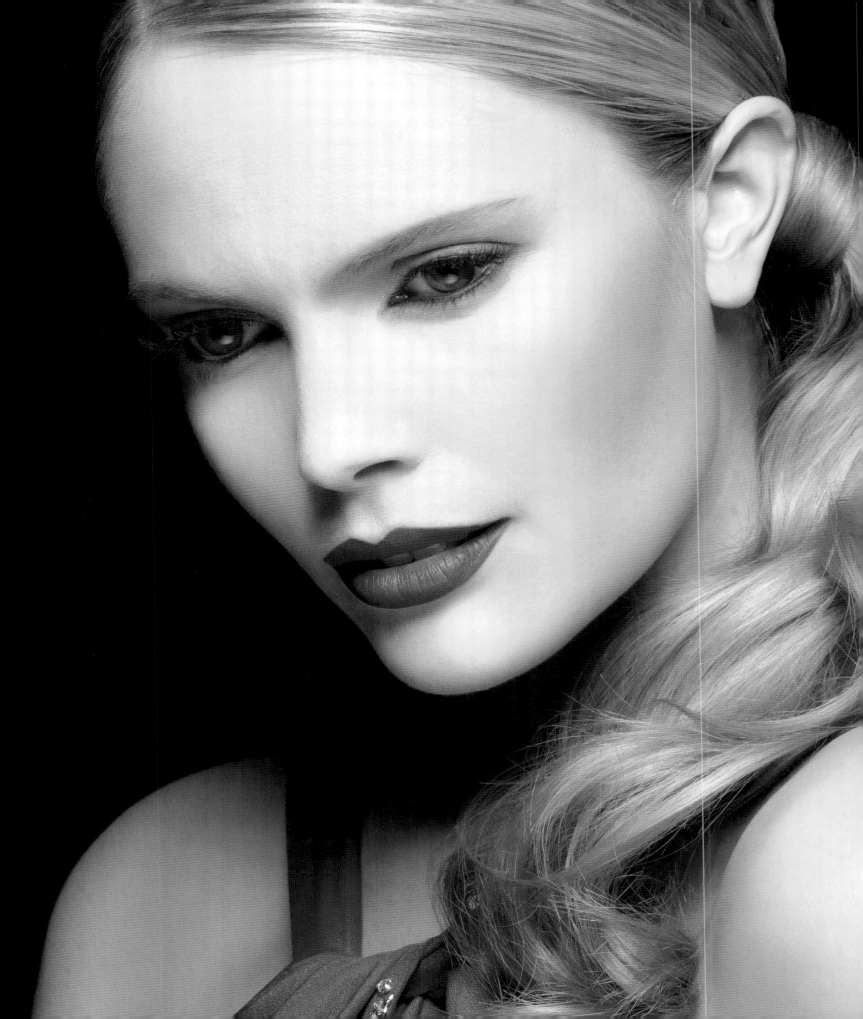

Eyes Tidy the brows and emphasize the arch. Pat a little concealer or primer over the eyelid to neutralize any redness. Apply pale beige or cream eyeshadow (**1**) over the lid from the lash line to the browbone, then blend a slightly darker neutral shade (**2**) into the socket crease. Using a gunmetal eye pencil (**3**), draw along the upper lash line, working the tip between the lashes for added volume. Draw just under the lower lashes and soften the line with a smudger. Curl the lashes and apply lengthening black mascara (**4**).

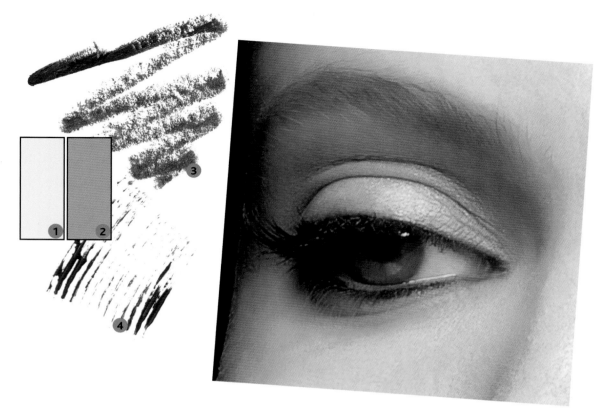

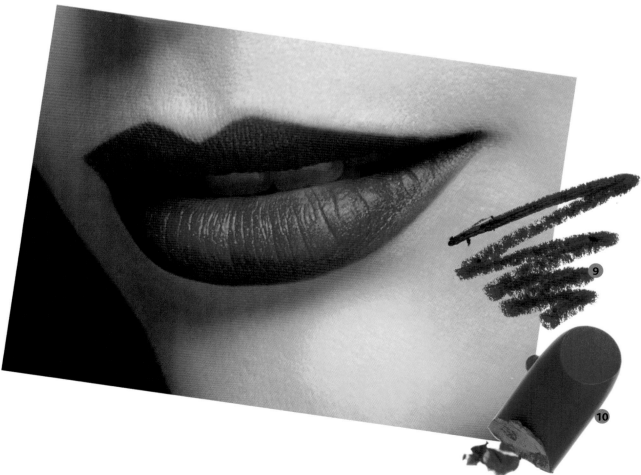

Lips Dab concealer around the lip area and over the lip itself – this removes any redness so that the line of the lips will be sharp and defined. Spend time drawing the perfect symmetrical outline with a red lip pencil (**9**) (see page 132). Fill in the colour with the pencil and smooth it out with a brush. Apply creamy scarlet lipstick (**10**) over the top, blot and reapply for a long-lasting finish.

HOW TO GET RED-CARPET READY

Face

» Cleanse and exfoliate thoroughly, apply a hydrating mask and a generous amount of moisturizer. Use a hydrating eye serum.

» To help keep make-up on and give skin a youthful glow, use an illuminating primer under foundation.

» A touch of highlighter on the points of the cheekbones and chin contours the face into a perfect oval.

» If there is likely to be flash photography, it's essential not to use too much powder. If you have oily skin, apply shimmer-free translucent powder only on the areas that catch the light, such as the bridge of the nose and tops of the cheekbones.

Eyes

» For eyeliner with staying power, draw a thin line along the roots of the upper lashes with a creamy pencil, then run over it with a fine pointed brush dipped in liquid liner. When it's dry, apply a little eyeshadow of the same colour on top.

» A dab of highlighter at the inner corner of the eyes opens them out.

Lips

» As lips are going to be strong, make sure they are flake-free and well moisturized.

Face Prep the face well and apply illuminating primer. Choose a foundation with a matte finish (**5**) and work it thoroughly into the skin. Apply concealer (**6**) where needed, then dust lightly with translucent powder (**7**). Create a natural glow by sweeping a little soft pink powder blush (**8**) onto the apples of the cheeks and blending it along the cheekbones.

dancing queen

KEY CONSIDERATIONS

» Glitter eyeshadow is a party look that is most flattering on young, wrinkle-free eyes. As a rule, the younger you are, the more you can use shimmer and glitter.

» There are plenty of subtler ways to introduce sparkle, which work on mature skin as well. Look for a pearlescent finish, which adds light without highlighting creases and wrinkles.

The perfect party look, glitter never fails to get girls in the mood to hit the dance floor. The inspiration is the heady days of disco, Studio 54 and 1970s glam rock, but toned down for a more refined interpretation.

Glitter shadow comes in various colours, but neutral metallics such as gold and silver are more understated. To wear glitter on your eyes, you need to have large eyelids that aren't hooded, otherwise the make-up will crease. If it won't work for you, there are other ways to bring a touch of shimmer to your look. And unless you're very young and a regular on the club scene, it's advisable to use glitter in moderation – it's easy to go more drag queen than dancing queen, so keep your look subtle.

'Apply glitter before making up the rest of your face and dust away any particles before applying foundation.'

VARIATIONS

» Make your own crème shimmer by mixing silver or gold loose powder with Vaseline. Apply with your finger or a brush up to the socket crease and then smudge beyond. Outline the inner rims and lash lines with black eyeliner.

» For a flash of metal, apply metallic liquid eyeliner along the upper lash line.

» Layer glitter gel eyeliner over dark eyeliner pencil.

TOP TIP

» A dusting of silver or gold eyeshadow on the inner corners of the eyes opens up close-set eyes.

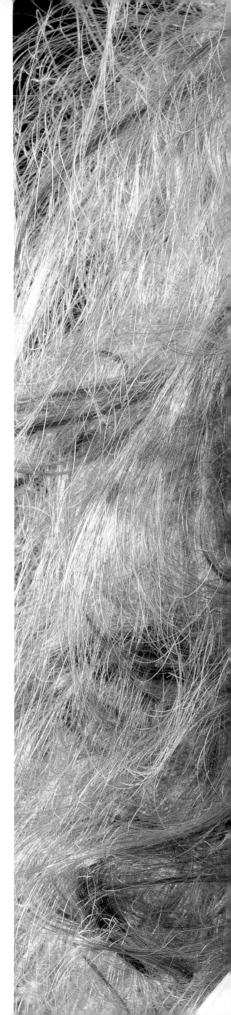

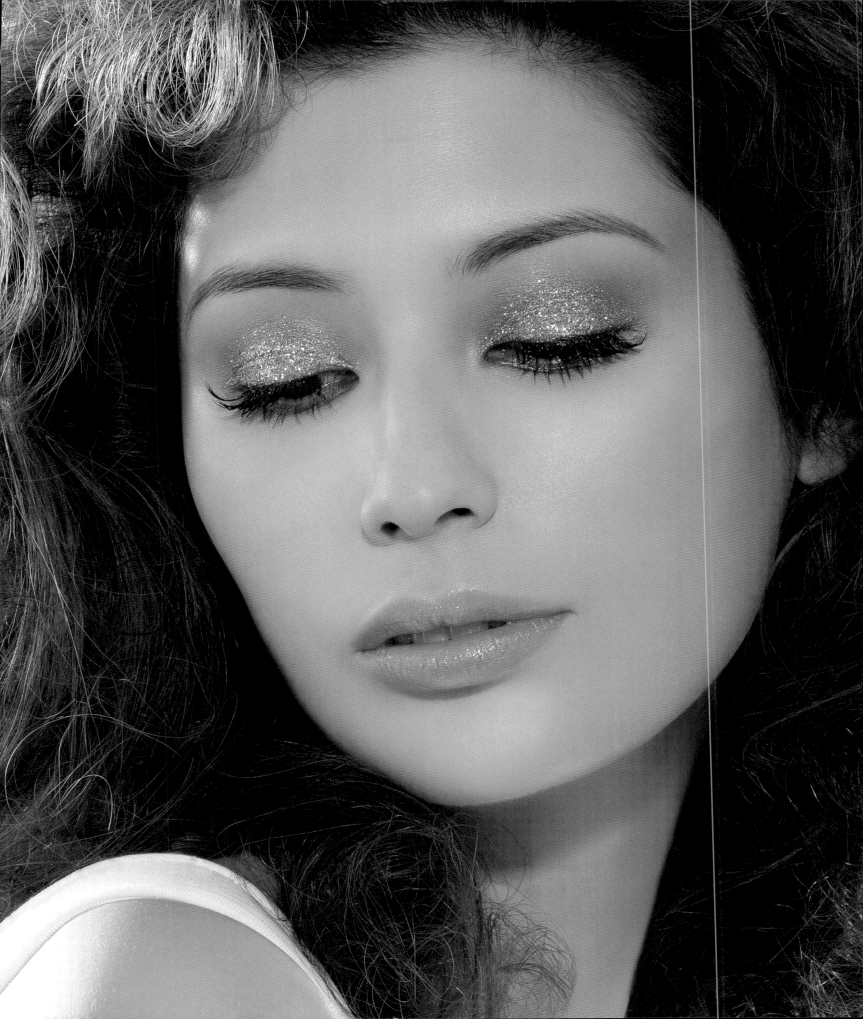

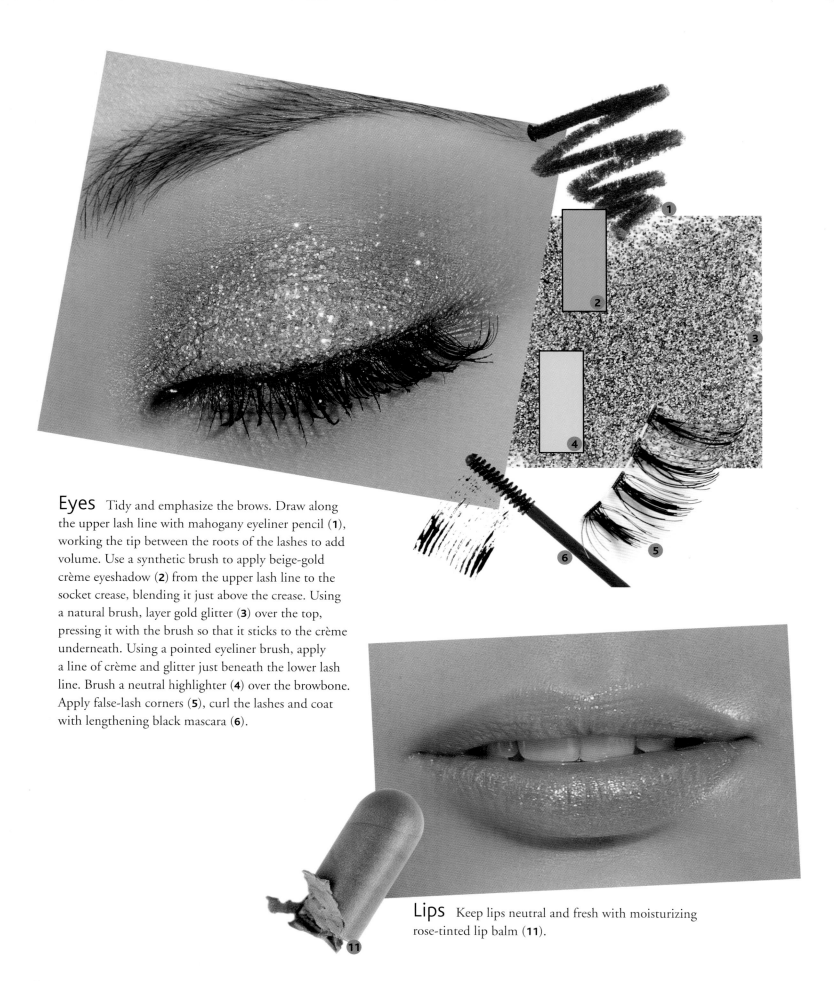

Eyes Tidy and emphasize the brows. Draw along the upper lash line with mahogany eyeliner pencil (**1**), working the tip between the roots of the lashes to add volume. Use a synthetic brush to apply beige-gold crème eyeshadow (**2**) from the upper lash line to the socket crease, blending it just above the crease. Using a natural brush, layer gold glitter (**3**) over the top, pressing it with the brush so that it sticks to the crème underneath. Using a pointed eyeliner brush, apply a line of crème and glitter just beneath the lower lash line. Brush a neutral highlighter (**4**) over the browbone. Apply false-lash corners (**5**), curl the lashes and coat with lengthening black mascara (**6**).

Lips Keep lips neutral and fresh with moisturizing rose-tinted lip balm (**11**).

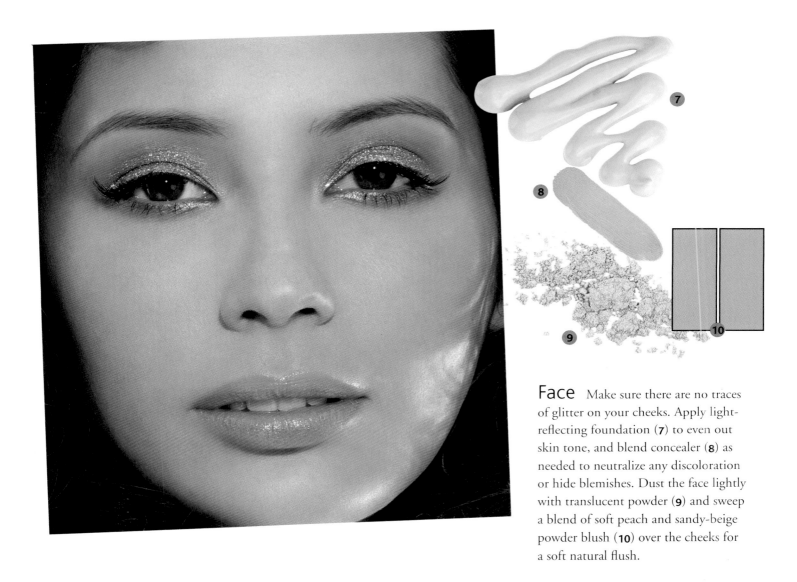

Face

Make sure there are no traces of glitter on your cheeks. Apply light-reflecting foundation (**7**) to even out skin tone, and blend concealer (**8**) as needed to neutralize any discoloration or hide blemishes. Dust the face lightly with translucent powder (**9**) and sweep a blend of soft peach and sandy-beige powder blush (**10**) over the cheeks for a soft natural flush.

GLITTER AND SHIMMER

Don't overdo the shimmer – if you have shine on your eyes, keep lips nude or matte; if lips are shimmering, keep eyes to a similar pearl finish and avoid shimmer on your face.

There are myriad shimmering shades for eyes, from all-out sparkle to subtle pearl. Try before buying, as shades that seem subtle in the palette can be more sparkly on skin.

For day use soft shimmering shades as a wash across the lid or to highlight under the browbone, but save glitter and highly pigmented shimmer for night.

Subtle shimmering shades that work well on mature skin or for daytime glamour are: soft bronze, brown, gold, peach, purple and pearl.

Lightly shimmering highlighter gives the face definition and luminosity. If your skin tone is cool, opt for a silvery tone; if your skin tone is warm or olive, use a gold-based highlighter.

Shimmering lipsticks or glosses in nude or pale pink add freshness to the look, but frost finishes tend to look dated.

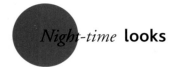

Night-time **looks**

big date

KEY CONSIDERATIONS

» On a date you want to look your most beautiful, with a clear, radiant complexion and your best features enhanced.

» Make-up should be feminine and sexy, but not overtly so.

» Most men prefer a natural look, so choose soft colours that work well with your skin tone and use shimmery, dewy textures that reflect the light.

The best advice I can give is to make sure you look like yourself, but your most gorgeous self. Spend time on your skin to ensure it's glowing with health, dewy and flawless. Exfoliate and moisturize your lips, and make sure your hands are soft with neat polished nails.

This look uses a palette of neutral colours to suit your skin tone, in textures that have a soft sheen or shimmer to reflect and bounce the light off your face, making you look vibrant and radiant. Eyes should have a doe-like quality, framed with lashes that are heavy, dark and irresistibly flirty.

TOP TIP
Pale to mid-toned lipsticks in satin or glossy textures will make lips look full and kissable.

VARIATIONS

» If you have cool pink-based porcelain or fair skin, try eyeshadows in shimmery champagne, mushroom or pearl grey, with soft pink lipstick.

» If you have warmer yellow-based olive skin, try peach, taupe or bronze eyeshadow, and lipstick with peach or orange tones.

» If you have dark skin, deeper colours work well – shimmery eyeshadow in soft plum, brown or burnt orange with lipstick in berry or plum tones.

'Knowing you look your best will give you the confidence to be yourself and let your personality sparkle.'

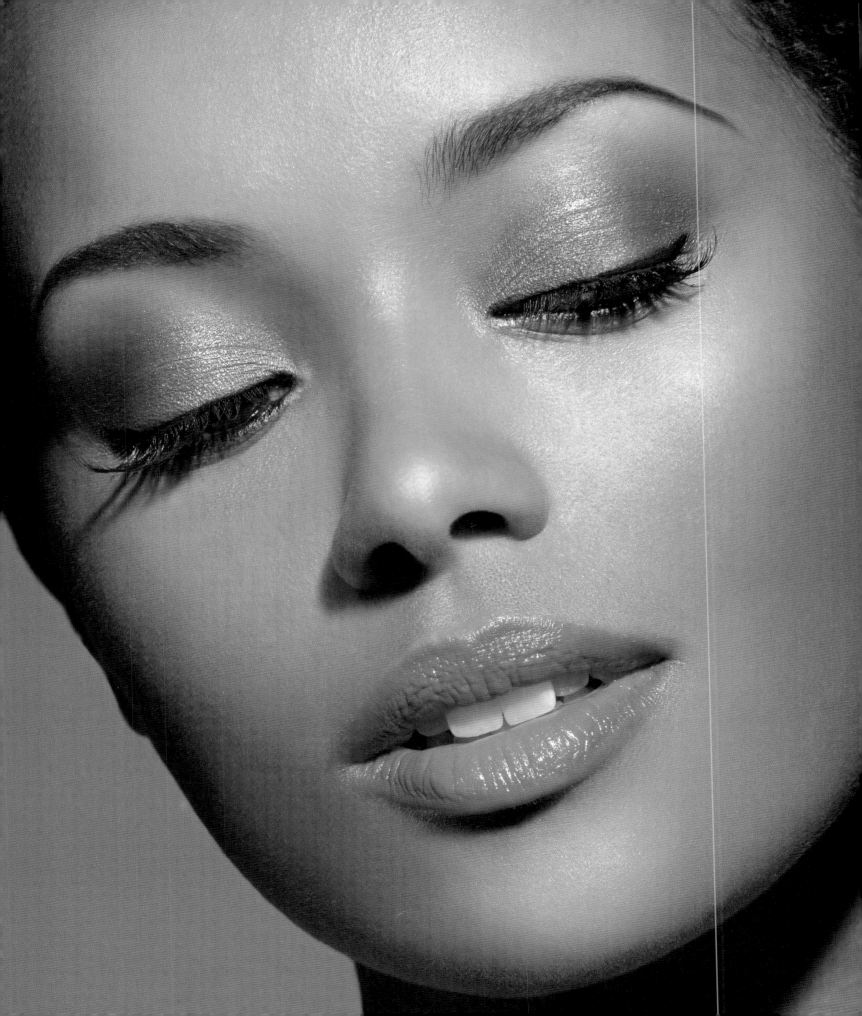

Eyes

Tidy and define the brows. Draw along the upper lash line with a black eyeliner pencil (**1**). Thicken the line gradually from the middle of the eyelid towards the outer corner of the eye, extending it slightly beyond the eye and curving it upwards to create a subtle flick. Draw along the inner rim of the lower lid to elongate the eye. Brush neutral beige eyeshadow (**2**) over the lid from the lash line to the browbone. Blend shimmery mocha eyeshadow (**3**) on top, working it from the lash line to the socket crease. For definition, blend plum eyeshadow (**4**) into the hollow of the socket, focusing on the outer corners. Using a fine eyeliner brush, apply a thin line of shimmery mocha shadow just under the roots of the lower lashes and blend a touch into the inner corners to open up the eyes. Apply false-lash corners (**5**), curl the lashes and apply lengthening black mascara (**6**).

Lips

Apply silky lipgloss in shell pink for a touch of soft colour and sheen.

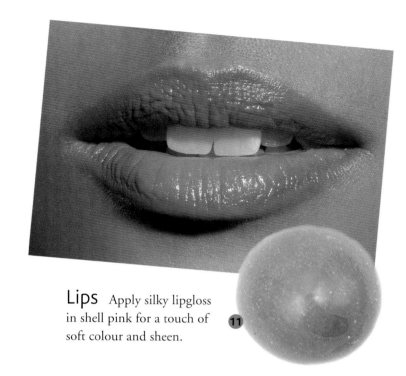

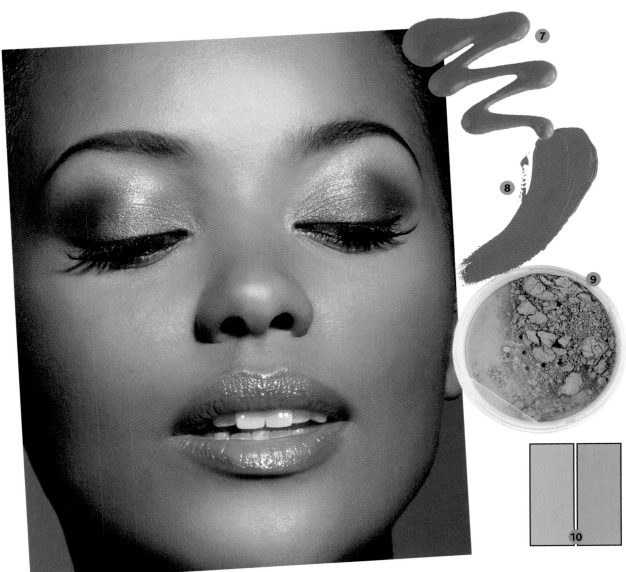

Face For a semi-matte finish, use light-reflecting liquid foundation (**7**) or mineral foundation if your skin is oily. Apply concealer (**8**) as needed to hide blemishes or discoloration. If you've used liquid foundation, dust with translucent powder (**9**) to set. Apply a blend of sandy-beige and pink powder blush (**10**) to the apples of the cheeks and blend along the cheekbones.

THE RULES

Most men aren't fans of too much make-up, so don't freak them out by using too much colour – save extreme looks for another occasion and aim for natural, feminine beauty.

That said, make-up should boost your confidence and express your personality, so don't tone down your look too much or you may not feel yourself.

Enhance your features. There should be lots of eye contact, so make your eyes big and seductive, with long dark lashes to flutter alluringly.

Lips should be kissable – smooth, soft and moisturized. Make them up to look full and pouty – pale to mid colours with a touch of sheen or non-sticky gloss fit the bill.

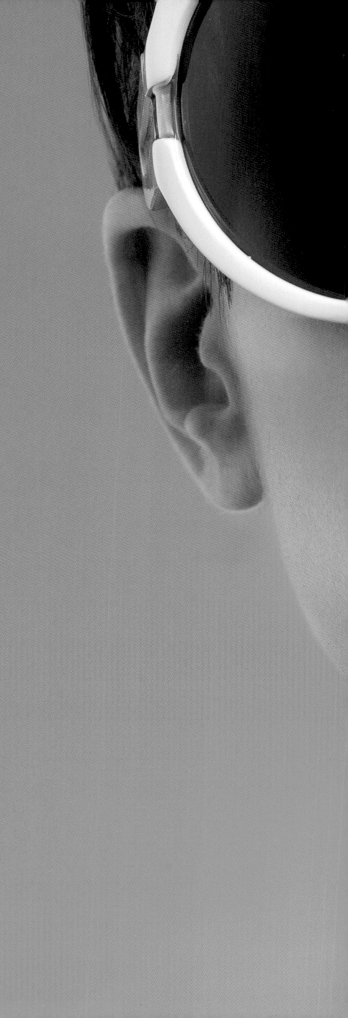

HOLIDAY

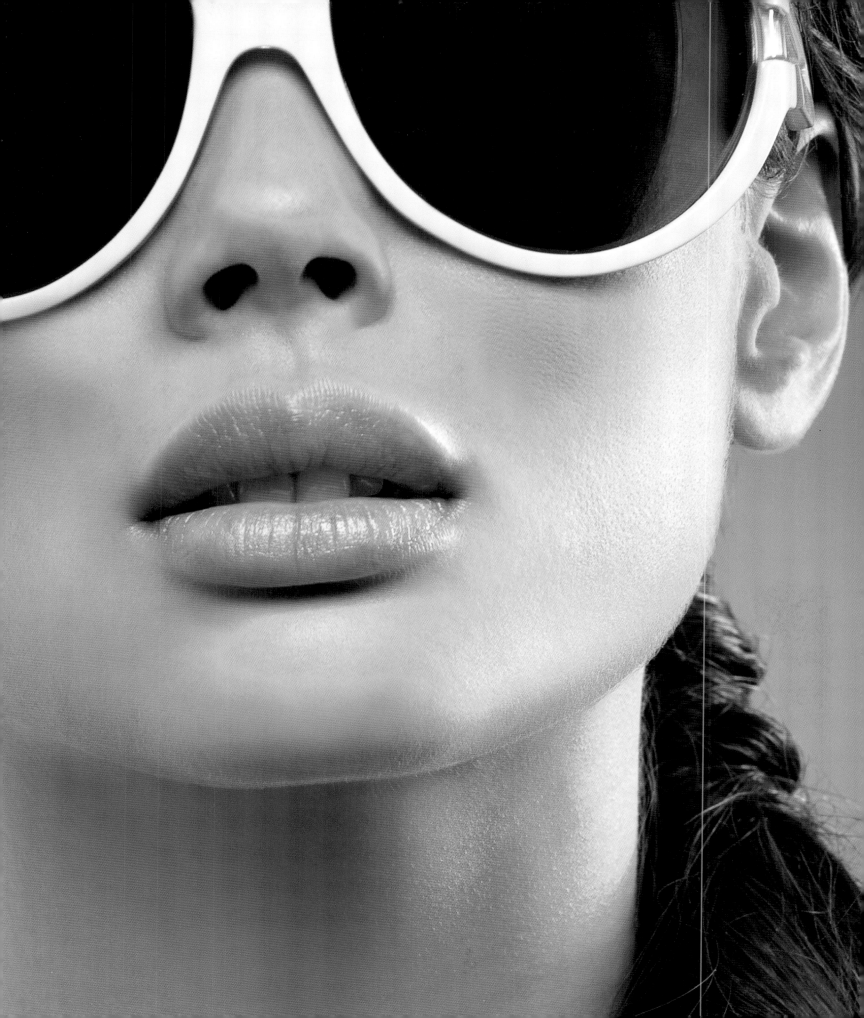

beach babe

KEY CONSIDERATIONS

» In the sun and heat, too much make-up will look unnatural and may clog or slide if you sweat, so go as bare as you dare and choose sheer tinted moisturizer over foundation.

» Use waterproof formulations and consider having your brows and lashes tinted.

» Protection is the most important thing – reapply sun cream and lip balm regularly.

Looking good on the beach can seem a challenging prospect, especially at the beginning of your holiday when it seems strange to bare so much flesh. Mix a little body shimmer into your sunscreen to prevent your skin from looking dull, and use make-up to define your eyes and add a healthy glow.

If you're likely to be on the beach all day, moisturize well and apply sunscreen, then either just use a touch of concealer under the eyes and around the nose to counteract redness, or apply tinted moisturizer or a complexion enhancer. Make sure the colour is very sheer so that it blends with your skin as it tans. Keep blotting tissues in your bag to get rid of shine. If you have tinted eyelashes, just apply clear mascara for definition and tone down any redness on the lid with eye primer. If you want to wear eyeshadow, keep it neutral and look for a long-lasting formulation. Wear a straw or fabric hat to shade your face and sunglasses to protect your eyes – the perfect way to look glamorous with minimal make-up.

VARIATIONS

Eyes

» Golden-toned eyeshadows complement a tan and open up the whole eye area.

» White pearlescent shadow contrasts with a tan and makes a great highlighter. Sweep it up to the browbones and line your eyes with a smoky brown pencil.

» Clear or brown mascara instead of black keeps the look natural.

Lips

» Warm pinks, bronzes, golds and beiges complement a golden skin colour.

» Frosted finishes are too wintry – go for a soft-touch gloss or sheer lipstick.

» Leave lipliner at home – it can look too strong.

TOP TIPS – BEFORE YOU GO

» You'll be less tempted to broil yourself if you're looking tanned to begin with. Fake tan is the answer, not a sunbed. A good fake tan should contain SPF, and some have added shimmer and moisturizers. Exfoliate beforehand, as this will help it go on more evenly and last longer.

» For low-maintenance beauty, have your eyebrows shaped and your lashes tinted.

» Bright nails look great with a tan, but natural nails that have been buffed to a shine are lower maintenance.

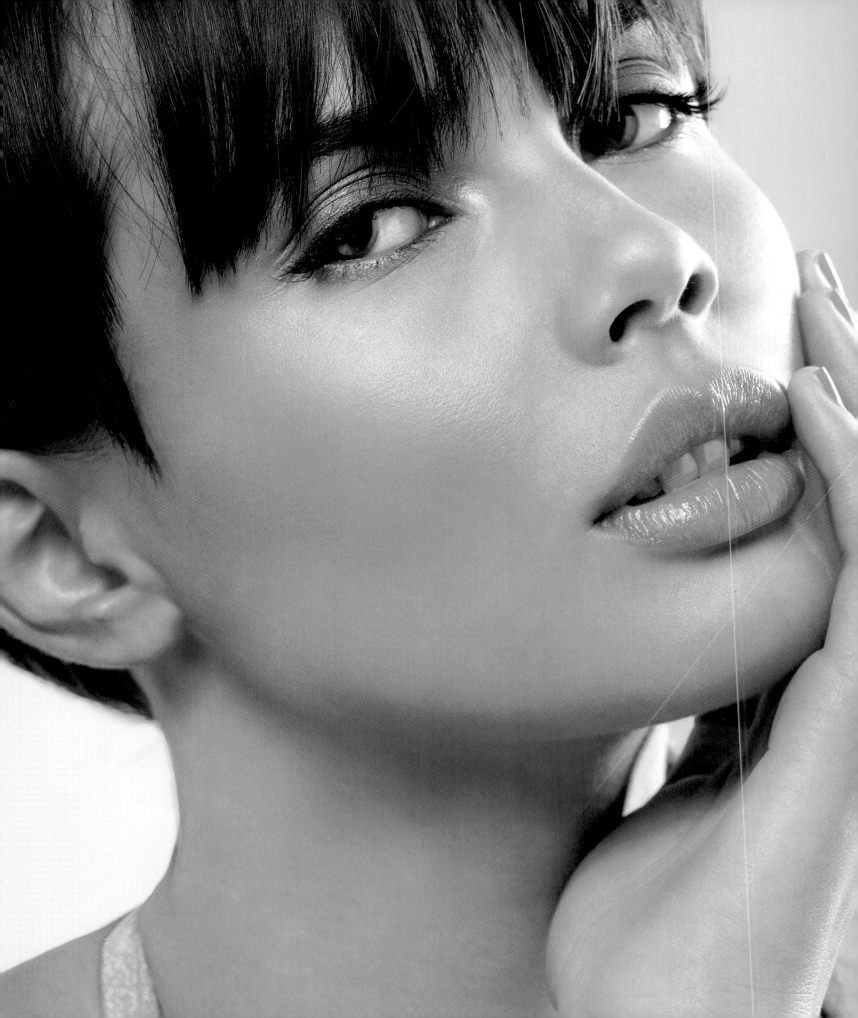

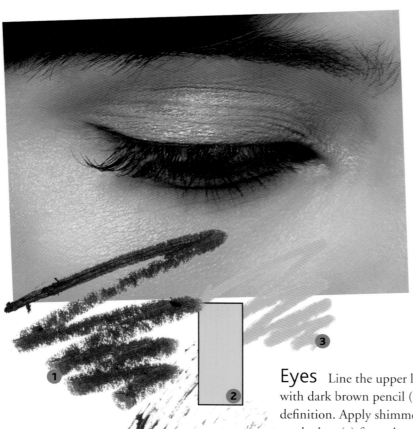

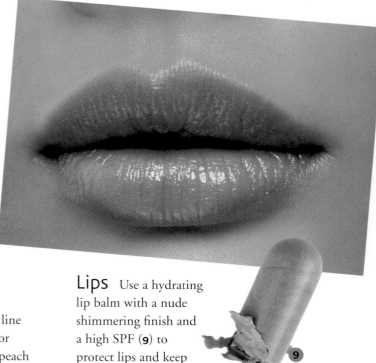

Eyes Line the upper lash line with dark brown pencil (**1**) for definition. Apply shimmery peach eyeshadow (**2**) from the upper lash line to the socket crease. Add a little shimmer under the lower lash line using gold eyeliner pencil (**3**). Apply dark brown waterproof mascara (**4**).

Lips Use a hydrating lip balm with a nude shimmering finish and a high SPF (**9**) to protect lips and keep them feeling moist despite sea spray and sun. Nude/brown tones are more flattering with a tan than red.

'Protect your skin with a moisturizing high-SPF sun cream (at least SPF 30 for your face) – UVA causes long-term damage and UVB causes sunburn, which can occur in less than 20 minutes' exposure to the sun.'

SWIMPROOF MAKE-UP

FACE Unless you need coverage, keep skin bare of make-up and just define the eyes. There are some very good waterproof foundations, but if you find them too heavy try gel bronzer, which is easy to apply evenly and won't come off until you cleanse.

EYES There's a big difference between 'water-resistant' – fine if you weep at the end of a movie – and 'waterproof', which can cope with a swim in the sea. Use waterproof eyeliners and mascaras, then touch up eyeshadow on the lid or highlighter under the browbone after your swim.

CHEEKS AND LIPS A lip stain is a good way to provide a healthy flush for both lips and cheeks without heavy make-up. After your swim, add a touch of lipgloss to lift the look and apply protective balm regularly.

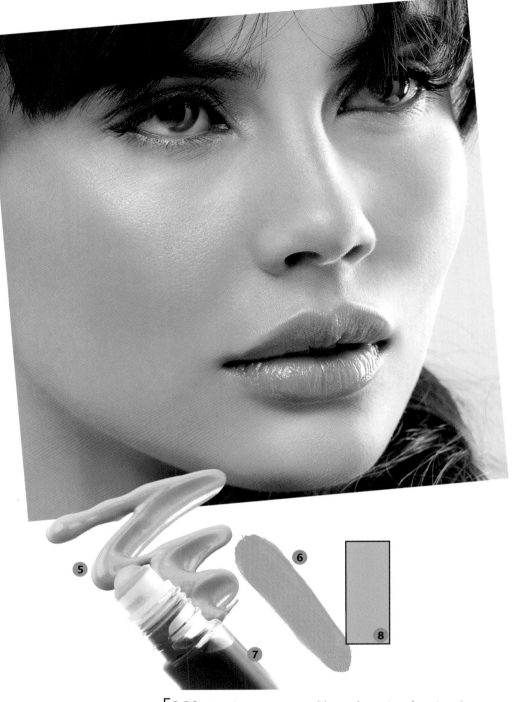

Sunburn make-up remedies

Despite your efforts to protect your skin, sometimes you stay out longer than expected or underestimate the power of the sun. Here's how to help your skin recover.

» Mix a little milk and cold water and apply with a muslin cloth to take down redness and cool the skin.

» Cocoa butter and aloe gel are excellent for preventing peeling. Cucumber creams are hydrating, while calendula ointment reduces inflammation.

» Gently pat in a creamy yellow-based concealer to neutralize redness. Don't use powder unless it is very fine.

» To cool down burnt eyelids, use a compress with milk and water or slices of cucumber, then apply a light hydrating gel. When the redness has died down, you can apply crème eyeshadow, a sweep of highlighter under the brow and clear mascara – keep make-up minimal, as removing it may be painful.

» Apply a moisturizing lip balm religiously, but avoid any containing menthol, which is painful on burnt lips.

Face Apply sunscreen and layer sheer tinted moisturizer on top (5), blending it well. Pat on concealer (6) as needed to cover blemishes or redness. Bring a natural flush to your cheeks by blending in pink cheek stain (7), which is water-resistant and will last longer than crème blush. If you need it, blend a little gold-toned highlighter or crème bronzer (8) onto the cheekbones, bridge of the nose, chin and temples.

BEACH TO BAR

After hours on the beach, try to find somewhere to wash your face in fresh water to remove sweat, dirt, sun cream and sea salt. If your skin is looking good, a touch of tinted moisturizer over cheeks or areas that tend to go red should be all you need, with a whip of bronzer for added glow. Redefine the eyes with smudgeproof eyeliner and use metallic bronze or gold eyeshadow to accentuate your sunkissed look. Add another coat of mascara, focusing on the roots to make lashes look thicker.

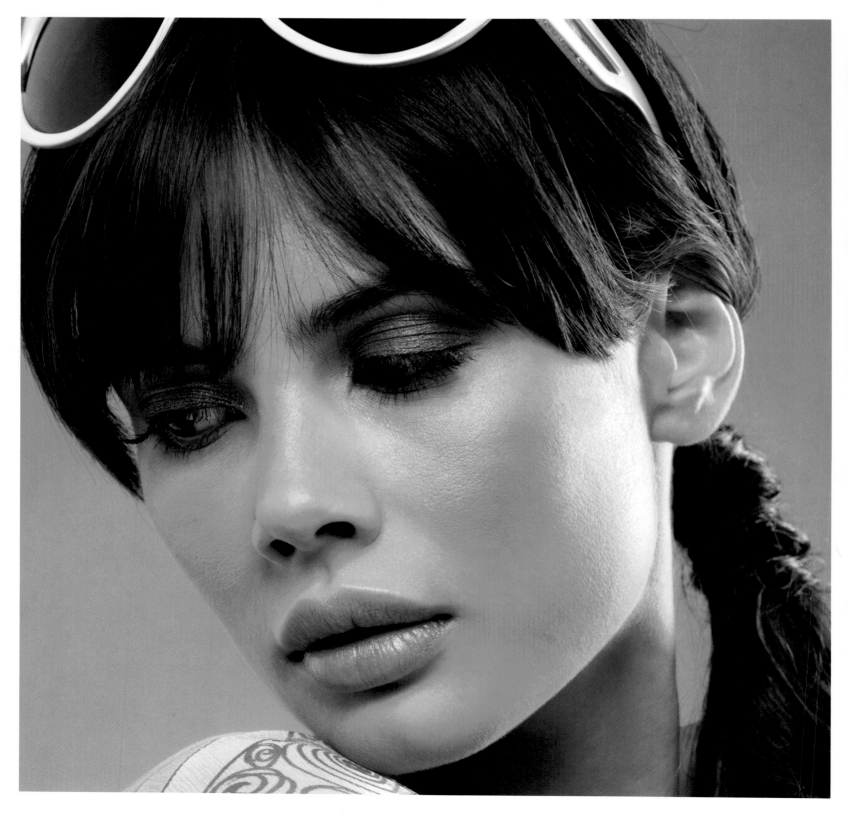

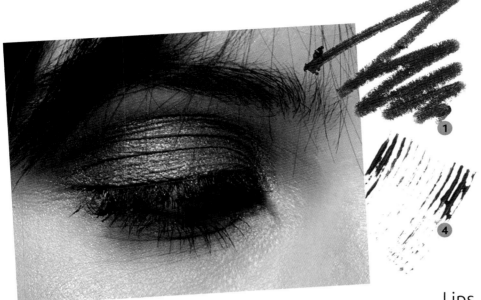

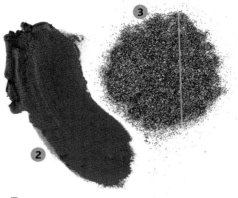

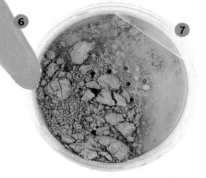

Eyes
Draw along the upper and lower lash line with black eyeliner pencil (**1**). Apply bronze crème eyeshadow (**2**) over the lid and layer with bronze metallic pigment (**3**). Apply black mascara (**4**) to define and thicken the lashes.

Face
Apply tinted moisturizer (**5**) and concealer (**6**) as needed, then lightly dust with a little translucent powder (**7**) before sweeping a little bronzer (**8**) over the cheekbones and temples.

Lips
Moisturize with nude lip balm (**9**), then add a layer of non-sticky nude or soft pink lipgloss (**10**).

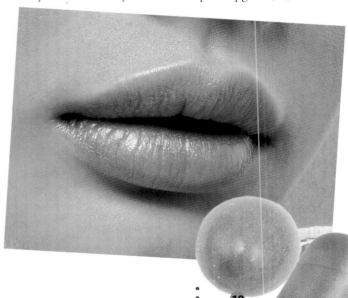

HOW TO PROLONG YOUR TAN

MOISTURIZE Skin can feel tight and dehydrated after a day in the sun, so apply an intensive moisturizer to nourish and soothe, leaving skin smooth, plumped and less likely to peel. Use a hydrating face mask to restore moisture and help repair damage. Aftersun lotion containing fake tan gives a subtle colour without being too orange.

MAKE-UP When your skin is tanned, your normal foundation can look like a pale mask. Use a foundation a few shades darker, or do without and use a tinted moisturizer or radiance crème for bare-faced shimmer.

BRONZER To revive a fading tan, apply a touch of bronzer on areas that naturally catch the sun. Powder bronzer can be brushed in a T-shape over the nose and forehead, with a little on the cheekbones, collarbones, décolletage and sides of the neck. For day use a light-reflecting crème bronzer. Body moisturizers with added gold give a light glow to arms and legs.

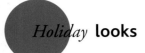

wintry and wonderful

KEY CONSIDERATIONS

» Cold weather is very drying, so use a richer face cream than usual and choose moisturizing and hydrating make-up formulations.

» The Snow Queen look relies on achieving a flawless, even complexion with a translucent quality.

» Eyes should be pale and iridescent, so white or silver metallic crème is ideal – crème eyeshadow is more moisturizing than powder.

» Lips need a gloss finish for an icy, shimmery look.

Whether you're going on a chic city break in chilly climes or wanting to looking pretty on the piste, the most important thing is to protect your skin from the drying and damaging effects of cold wind and winter sun. Prepare your skin in the run-up to your holiday by treating it to a hydration-boosting face mask and extra-rich cream to build up its defences against moisture loss.

The inspiration for this beautiful, icy, fairytale look is pure White Witch, straight from the set of *Narnia*, with iridescent metallic white eyeshadow, shimmery cool-pink glossy lips and matte translucent skin. The whole effect is magical, frosty and ethereal.

VARIATIONS

» Pure white metallic eyeshadow looks magical on anyone with naturally pale skin, but if your complexion is darker you can achieve a similar ethereal quality by using metallic crème, silver or gunmetal eyeshadow and liner.

» For mid-tone and warmer skin, go for pale peachy blush and lipstick instead of cool blue-based pinks; for dark skin, choose deep plum shades.

'If your skin is dry, choose a moisturizing liquid foundation and don't use powder.'

TOP TIPS – BEFORE YOU GO

» Use a gentle exfoliator to lift away dead skin cells and reveal brighter skin beneath. Look for ingredients such as green tea and aloe to calm and protect the skin, or essential oils to soften and condition.

» Give your skin a moisture boost with a hydrating mask, and use a hydrating serum under your daily moisturizer and a really rich cream at night.

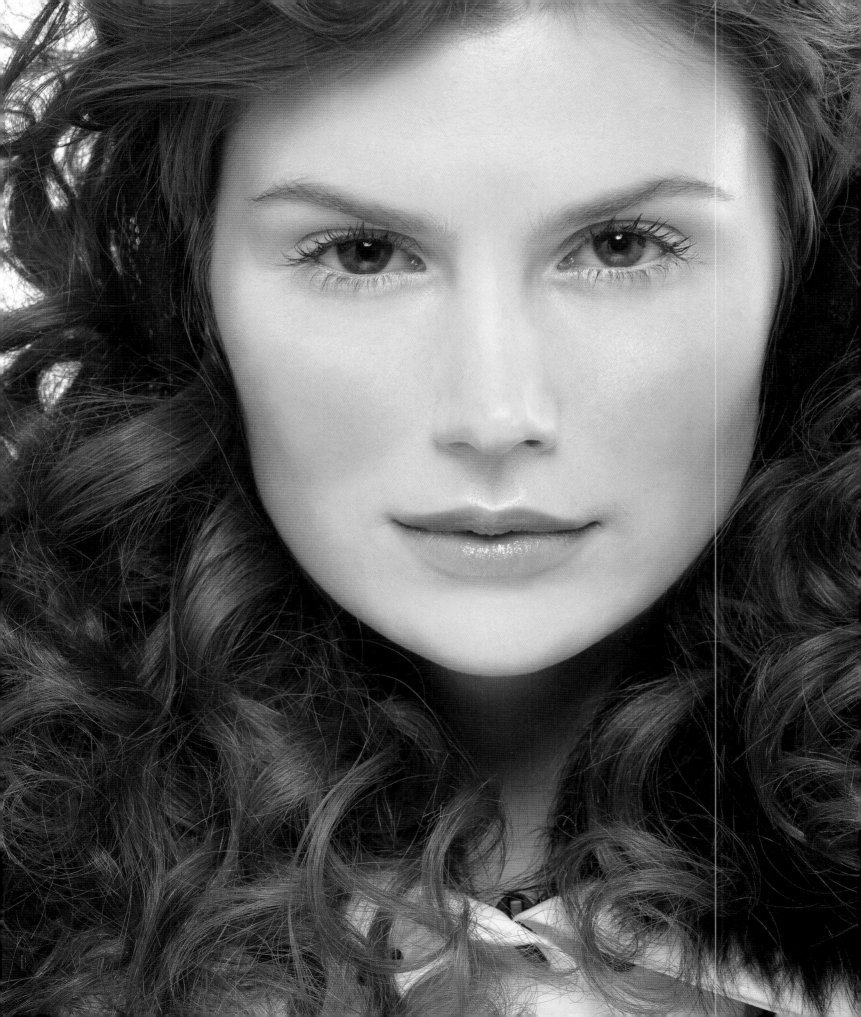

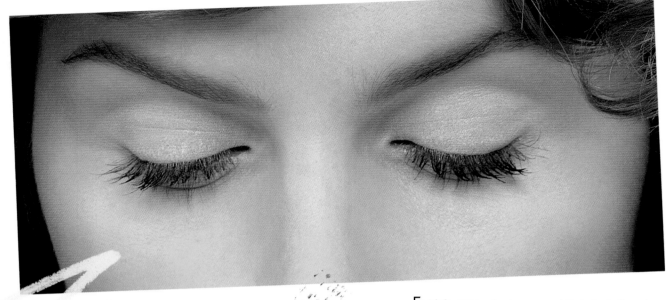

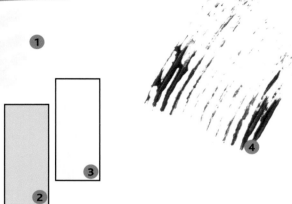

Eyes
Tidy the brows and lightly define the shape. Pat a little concealer or eye primer over the lids and at the corners of the eyes if necessary to neutralize any redness. Using a white eyeliner pencil (**1**), outline the eyes all the way around, including the inner corners, and draw along the inner rim of the lower lids. Apply a wash of cream matte powder eyeshadow (**2**) over the lids from the lash line to the browbone. Using a synthetic brush, apply frosty metallic crème eyeshadow (**3**) over the lids, blending it from the lash line to the socket crease. Apply lengthening brown mascara (**4**) to the upper lashes only.

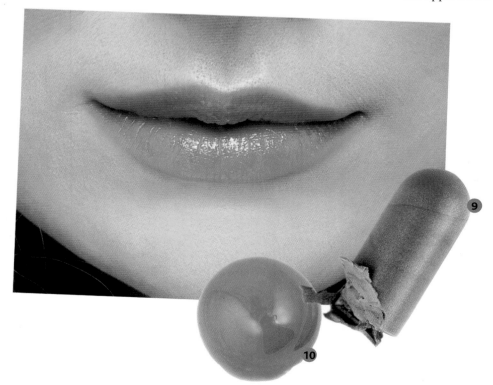

Lips
Moisturize and protect the lips with hydrating balm (**9**), then apply candy-pink lipgloss (**10**) for a cool glassy finish.

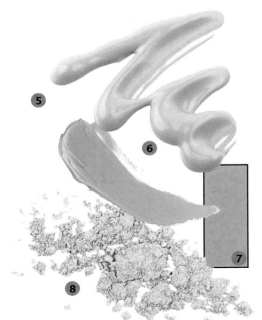

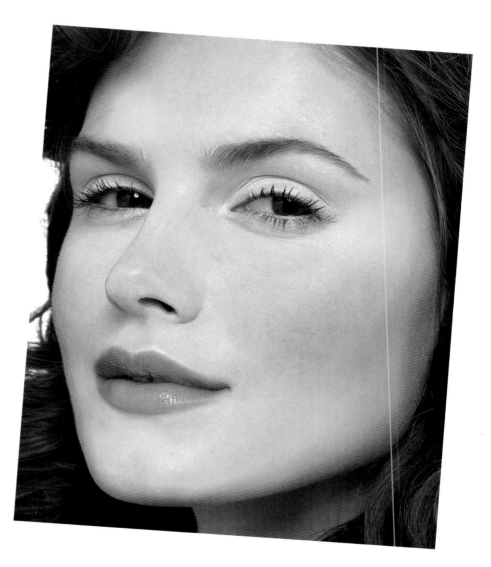

Face

Use a rich moisturizer to form a protective barrier against the drying effects of cold weather. Apply moisturizing radiance-boosting liquid foundation (**5**) to even out skin tone and give an iridescent quality. Pat in concealer (**6**) where needed to hide any blemishes and neutralize redness, which can be exacerbated by cold weather. Blend cool pink crème blush (**7**) over the cheekbones for a natural-looking flush. Dust the face with ultra-fine translucent powder (**8**) for a velvety smooth finish.

WINTER SUN It may be cold, but when you're out in the winter sun it's as important as ever to wear products with the right level of protection for your skin – for both face and hands – especially if you're skiing or by water.

High SPF sunscreens often contain mineral blocks, which tend to sit visibly on the skin. While these may be the best option for very sensitive skin, you need to blend foundation twice as carefully to ensure proper absorption.

Look for SPF 25 in your moisturizer. If you are going outside in freezing temperatures, an oil-based moisturizer will be best, even if your skin is prone to oiliness – water can freeze on the face, causing a burning sensation.

As the delicate eye area needs only light moisturization, use your usual eye cream, but make sure you cover well with a foundation or concealer that contains a high SPF.

While there's no harm in layering products with SPF in them, they don't add together – a moisturizer with SPF 15 and a foundation with SPF 10 gives you SPF 15, not 25.

As lips have no oil glands, they easily become chapped by the cold as well as burnt by the sun. Petroleum-based products form a barrier that can actually be more drying in the long term. Instead, look for natural balms.

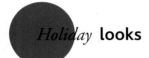

Holiday **looks**

country life

KEY CONSIDERATIONS

» The look is fresh and wholesome, as though you have a healthy glow from being out in the fresh air hiking or horse riding.

» Define the eyes but keep to a colour palette of earthy neutrals.

» Use creamy moisturizing formulations on the lips.

» Make-up should be long-lasting so that it stays the course while you're outdoors being active.

VARIATIONS

» For eyes, try moss greens, muddy browns, heathery purples, mushroom or stone.

» Lips can be nude or shades of soft brown or berry.

On a weekend in the country, the last thing you want to think about is applying full make-up and creating a 'look'. Make-up needs to be understated and simple, giving the impression that you're hardly wearing any and haven't made a huge effort. Now is the time to kick back and relax, exchanging your work wardrobe for country casuals and swapping your stilettos for wellies or walking shoes.

That said, you still want to look well-groomed and as gorgeous as ever with a clear, fresh complexion and defined eyes and lips. The emphasis is on longevity – when you're hiking up a hill or are caught in a shower, you don't want your make-up to slide or your mascara to run, so choose long-lasting waterproof formulations.

'Leave bright shades in town and keep colours on the face neutral and earthy or fresh and natural.'

TOP TIP

Start out wearing a creamy lipstick, but carry a tinted lip balm to refresh the colour throughout the day – it's easy to apply without a mirror or brush and will keep your lips hydrated.

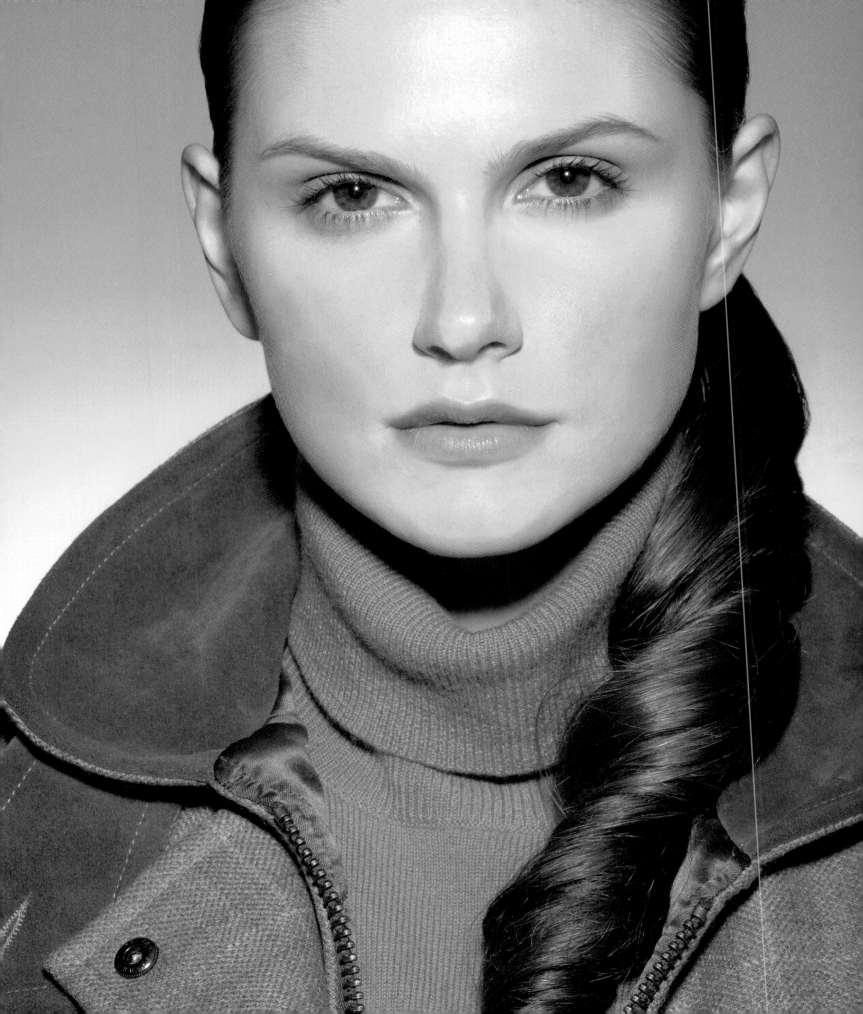

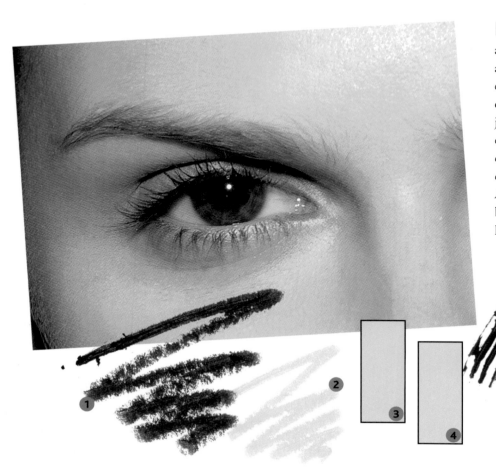

Eyes
Tidy the brows and use a brow pencil and powder to softly define their shape. Draw along the upper lash line with earthy-brown eyeliner pencil (**1**). For a brightening effect, draw along the inner rim of the lower lid and just underneath the lashes with flesh-toned eyeliner pencil (**2**). Using a pale caramel eye crayon with a subtle shimmer (**3**), fill in the eyelid from the lash line to the socket crease. Apply a neutral beige highlighter (**4**) on the browbone. Coat the lashes with dark brown lengthening mascara (**5**).

Lips
Apply pink lipstick (**10**) using a brush to press the colour into the lips for a long-lasting finish. Choose a creamy hydrating formula to keep the lips moisturized.

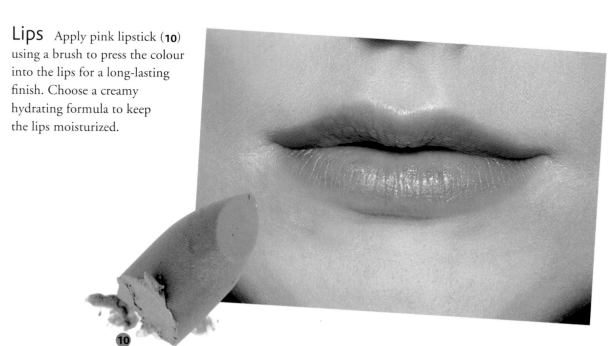

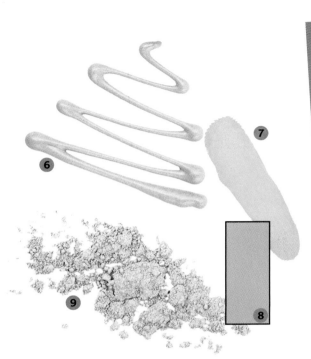

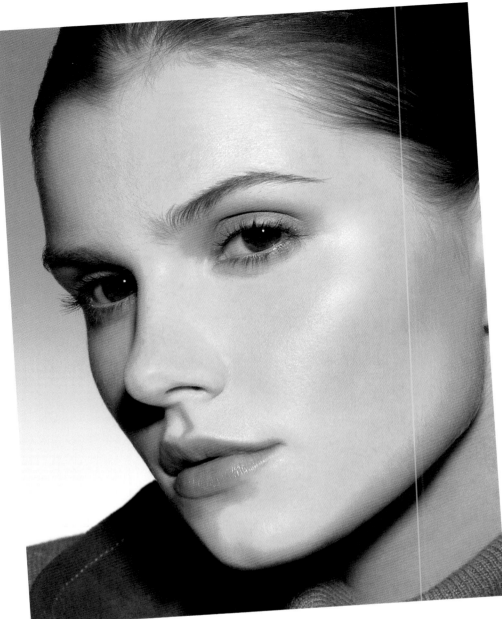

Face

Moisturize well to keep the skin hydrated and protected. Even out skin tone with matte foundation (**6**) and apply concealer (**7**) where needed to neutralize redness and hide any blemishes. Blend soft pink crème blush (**8**) onto the cheeks for a natural 'outdoor' flush. Lightly dust the face with ultra-fine translucent powder (**9**) to set the make-up.

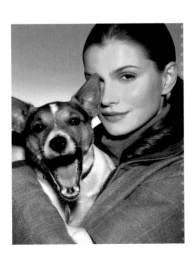

TOP TIPS FOR A FRESH-FACED GLOW

» Take inspiration from the landscape and opt for soft browns and taupes on the eyes.

» Use very little foundation – just enough to cover any redness or blemishes – or use tinted moisturizer and concealer.

» Use warm-toned blushes, such as shades of taupe or peach – nothing too red.

» Make sure brows are groomed but not heavily defined, and choose a mascara that lengthens the lashes rather than thickening them.

» Keep lips hydrated in natural colours, such as soft pinks and beige.

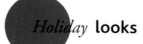
Holiday **looks**

frequent flyer

KEY CONSIDERATIONS

» Choose hydrating make-up to help prevent the skin from drying out – light liquid or crème formulations are more moisturizing than powders.

» Keep make-up minimal and focus on products that will brighten the skin and counter signs of flight fatigue.

» If you're being met at the airport or going straight to a meeting, travel light with two-in-one products and make sure you can apply them easily without brushes.

Whenever you're travelling, the make-up that you wear and take with you will depend on where you're going and for how long, as well as the duration of the flight and what you'll be doing when you land.

Long-haul flights are incredibly dehydrating, with the inactivity slowing down circulation and the dry atmosphere leaving skin feeling tight and uncomfortable. You may want to sleep, so keep make-up to a minimum, apply moisturizer and lip balm, and drink plenty of water.

Even short flights take their toll on the skin, while early starts and hanging around at airports can leave you looking as tired as you feel. If you travel for work, you may have to go straight to a meeting, so you'll need to apply quick and easy make-up to freshen your look and make you presentable.

'Pack facial wipes, moisturizer and essential make-up in your hand luggage to use during the flight or before landing.'

TOP TIPS FOR TRAVELLING LIGHT

» Decant your skincare products and sunscreen into travel-size containers.

» Instead of taking a separate moisturizer and foundation, try a tinted moisturizer containing SPF with a concealer to cover any imperfections.

» Take blotting tissues instead of powder to remove any excess oil from your face.

» If you use natural colour on the eyes, use the powders from your brow kit, or vice versa, rather than taking two compacts.

» Instead of a separate lipstick and blush, opt for a combined lip and cheek tint.

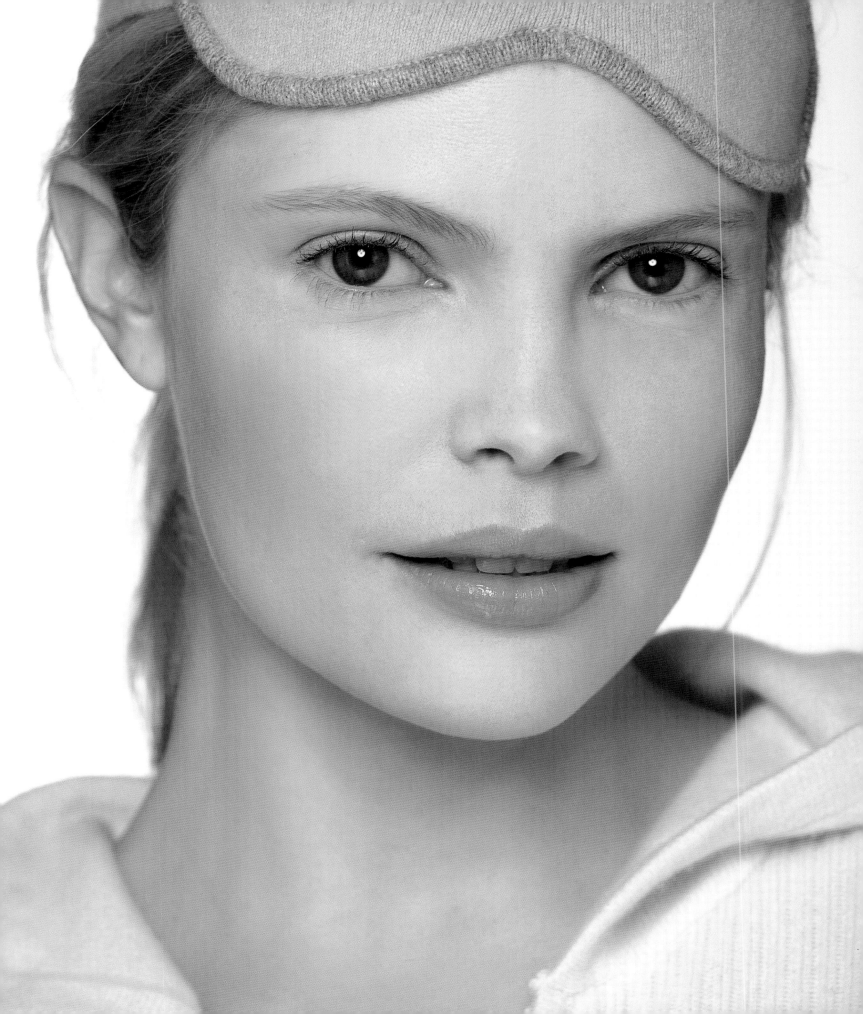

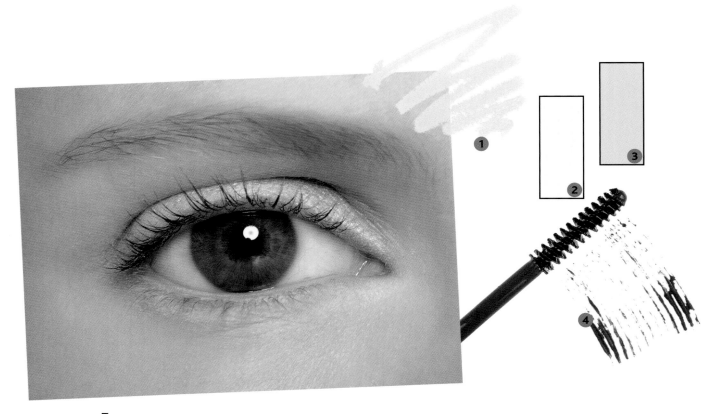

Eyes Neutralize any redness by patting a little concealer or eye primer over the eyelids. Using flesh-toned eyeliner pencil (**1**), draw along the inner rim and lash line of the lower lids to make the eyes look brighter. Apply a wash of subtly shimmering pearl eyeshadow (**2**) over the eyelids from the upper lash line to the browbone. Define the socket crease with a shimmering caramel eye crayon (**3**). Define the upper lashes with dark brown lash tint (**4**).

Lips Keep lips well moisturized with hydrating rose-tinted lip balm (**8**).

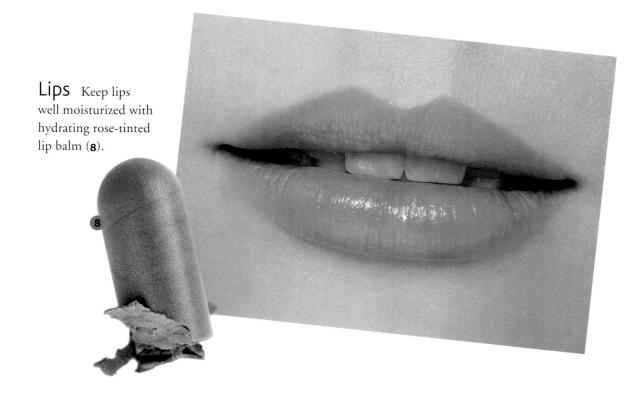

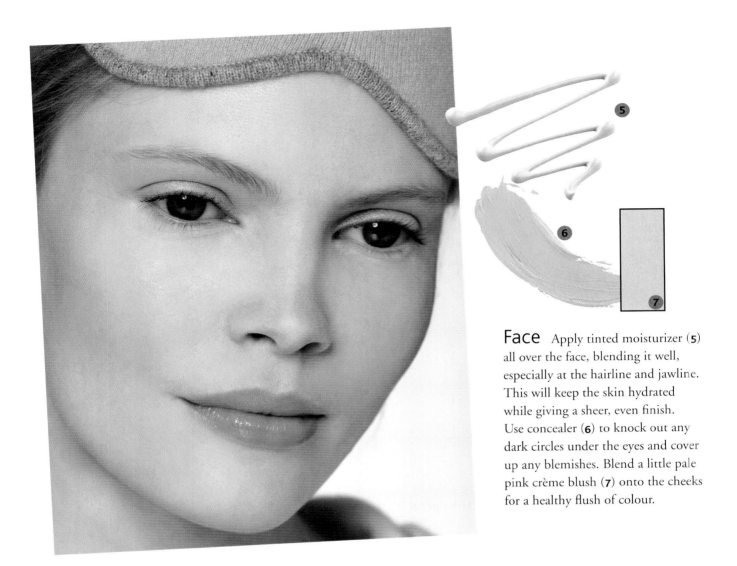

Face Apply tinted moisturizer (**5**) all over the face, blending it well, especially at the hairline and jawline. This will keep the skin hydrated while giving a sheer, even finish. Use concealer (**6**) to knock out any dark circles under the eyes and cover up any blemishes. Blend a little pale pink crème blush (**7**) onto the cheeks for a healthy flush of colour.

Pre-flight preparation

1 Use a deep-cleanser to make sure skin is really clean.

2 Exfoliate to remove dead skin cells.

3 Moisturize as normal.

4 Apply a light foundation base for the airport and a coat of mascara. Opt for crème make-up formulations, as they will be quicker to remove on the plane and won't dehydrate your skin.

5 Use a stain or a crème blush.

Mid-flight survival tips

1 Keep skin hydrated by drinking plenty of water.

2 Wipe away any make-up.

3 Apply a hydrating eye gel. You can also apply a clear face mask for extra hydration.

4 Use a wax-based lip balm to seal in moisture.

5 Use a hydrating facial spray or a moisturizer with soothing ingredients, such as aloe and calendula.

6 Avoid dehydrating salty foods, fizzy drinks and alcohol.

7 Use eye drops to stop eyes drying out.

Make-up for landing

1 Moisturize the skin.

2 Apply a little liquid foundation to even out the skin tone.

3 Use a lengthening mascara.

4 Add a touch of crème blush for a fresh-faced look.

5 When you arrive at your destination, have a warm bath with Epsom salts – it eases stress and flushes out toxins.

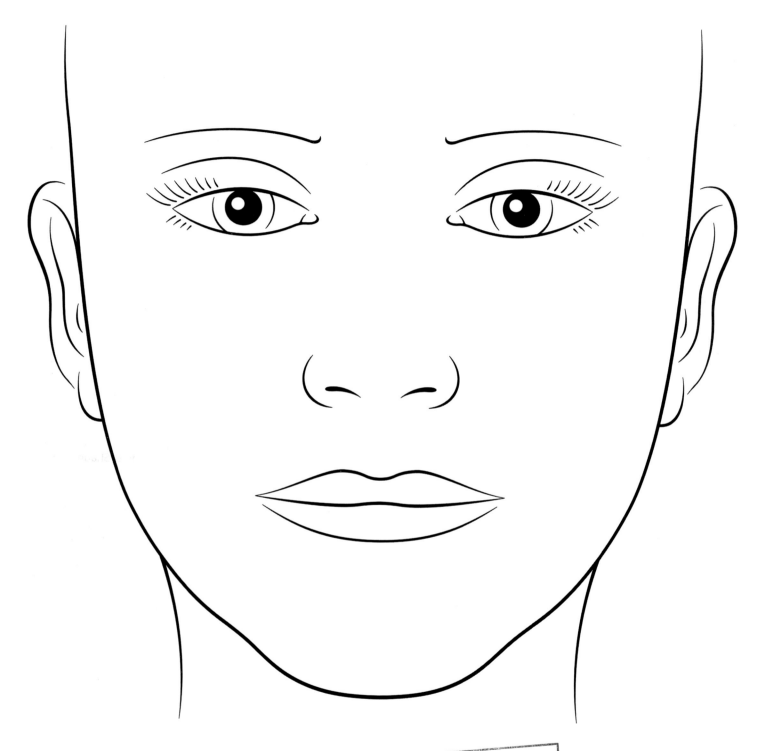

FACE MAP

Photocopy the face map above and use it to design your own make-up looks. Draw on your ideal eyebrow shape and be bold trying out different combinations of colours and textures for eyes, cheeks and lips.

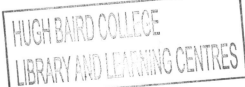

Jemma's favourite ...

Facial skincare products

Cleansers
Liz Earle Cleanse & Polish Hot
   Cloth Cleanser
La Roche Posay Effaclar
Lancôme Crème Radiance

Eye make-up removers
Dior Duo Magique Duo-Phase
   Eye Makeup Remover
L'Oréal De-Maq Expert

Exfoliators
Kate Somerville ExfoliKate
   Intensive Exfoliating Treatment
MAC Microfine Refinisher

Day moisturizers
Sarah Chapman Dynamic
   Defence SPF 15
Estée Lauder DayWear Plus
   SPF 15

Facial SPFs
La Roche Posay Anthelios XL
   SPF 50+
Jurlique Sun Lotion SPF 30+
Clinique Super City Block SPF 40
Aloe Gator SPF 40+ Gel
Elave Daily Skin Defence SPF 30+

Night moisturizers
Sarah Chapman Overnight Facial
Crème de la Mer

Eye creams
Zelens Intensive Triple Action
   Eye Cream
Yon Ka Phyto-Contour Eye
   Firming Cream

Hydrating mask
Sisley Express Flower Gel Mask

Facial oils/serums
Estée Lauder Advanced
   Night Repair
ILA Rose Oil
Dr Hauschka Normalising
   Day Oil

Body products

Hand cream
Elave Dermocosmetics Hand
   Treatment

Body moisturizers
La Roche-Posay Lipikar Body Milk
Soap & Glory Righteous Butter

Body shimmer
JK Jemma Kidd Show Stopper
   Year Round Body Glow

Make-up and tools

Eyes

Brow Kit
Jemma Kidd Make Up School
   Brow Kit

Eye pencil
Jemma Kidd Make Up School
   Define Stay-Put Eyeliner

Liquid eyeliners
Bobbi Brown Long Wear Gel
   Liner
MAC Fluidline

Powder eyehadows
MAC
Illamasqua
Chanel

Crème eyeshadows
Clinique Touch Tint for Eyes
Bobbi Brown Long-Wear Cream
   Shadow

Lash curler
Shu Uemura

Mascara
Dior Diorshow Blackout Mascara

Face

Primer
Jemma Kidd Make Up School
   Skin Rescue Bio Complex Veil

Tinted moisturizer
Laura Mercier Oil Free Tinted
   Moisturizer

Liquid foundations
Jemma Kidd Make Up School
   Light-As-Air
Make Up Forever High Definition
Chanel Vitalumière
Dior Diorskin Nude

Mineral foundations
Jane Iredale
Jemma Kidd Make Up School
   Mineral Tint SPF 20

Loose powder
Laura Mercier Secret Brightening
   Powder

Undereye concealers
Dior Skinflash
MAC Moisture Cover

Skin illuminator
JK Jemma Kidd Mannequin Skin
   Complexion Enhancer

Complexion enhancers
By Terry Eclat De Teint
Jemma Kidd Make Up School
   Dewy Glow Radiance Crème

Blemish concealer
Laura Mercier Secret
   Camouflage

Highlighters
JK Jemma Kidd i-Design in Elle
MAC Vanilla

Powder blushes
Shu Uemura
Nars

Crème blushes
Bobbi Brown Pot Rouge
Kevyn Aucoin

Bronzer
Guerlain Terracota

Cheek and lip stain
Jemma Kidd Make Up School
   Rosy Glow Lip & Cheek Tint

Lips

Lip balms
Sisley Nutritive Lip Balm
La Roche Posay Ceralip Lip
   Repair Cream

Lipliner
Jemma Kidd Make Up School
   Shape & Shade

Lipsticks
Guerlain Kiss Kiss (cream)
Revlon Matte (matte)
RMK Irresistible Lips (sheer)

Lipgloss
JK Jemma Kiss Lip ID Color
   Adapt Lip Gloss

Nails

Nail varnishes
Revlon Nail Enamel
OPI

Organic Make-up and Skincare Brands

Aesop
Aveda
Dr Hauschka – for foundation
   and bronzer

Elave
Green People – for lipstick
Living Nature – for mascara
Nvey Eco
Origins
Ren
The Organic Pharmacy
There Must Be A Way – for lip
crème

Brands and products for Problem Skin

Clinique Pore Minimizer
Clinique Redness Solutions
Coverblend – cosmetic
camouflage
Covermark – cosmetic
camouflage
Dermablend – cosmetic
camouflage
Dr Hauschka Rose Day Cream –
for sensitive rosacea-prone skin
Elave – for sensitive skin and
sufferers of dermatitis,
psoriasis and eczema
Prescriptives – for custom-blend
foundation and powder
Proactiv – for acne-prone skin

Treatments

London
Aglaia Hernandez Kortis at
Natureworks – for massage
Sarah Chapman – for facials
Spa NK
Strip Waxing Bar
Urban Retreat Spa at Harrods
Vanda Serrador at Urban Skin –
for facials and body treatments

New York
Ashley Javier Parlor – for hair
cut and colour
Bliss Spa
Lily's Nail Bar

Beverly Hills
Beverly Hills Hotel Spa

Stockists

*The products listed above can
all be purchased from on-line
retailers as well as most large
department stores. Check out
the websites below.*

For Jemma Kidd Make Up
School products, visit
www.spacenk.co.uk
+44 (0)20 8740 2085

For Jemma Kidd JK
products, visit
www.asos.com (UK)
www.target.com (USA)

For information on
professional make-up courses
and non-professional make-up
workshops, visit
www.jemmakidd.com
+44 (0)844 800 2636

Aesop
www.beautyexpert.co.uk
Aloe Gator
www.extremehorizon.com
Aglaia Hernandez Kortis
+44 (0)20 7629 2927
Ashley Javier Parlor
www.ashleyjavierparlor.com
Aveda
www.aveda.co.uk
Beverly Hills Hotel Spa
www.thebeverlyhillshotel.com/
fitness_spa/index.html
Bliss Spa
www.blissworld.com
Bobbi Brown
www.bobbibrown.co.uk
By Terry
www.byterry.com
Chanel

www.chanel.com
Clinique
www.clinique.co.uk
Coverblend
www.neostrata.com
Covermark
www.covermark.com
Crème de la Mer
www.cremedelamer.co.uk
Dermablend
www.dermablend.co.uk
Dior
www.dior.com
Dr Hauschka
www.drhauschka.co.uk
Elave
www.elave.co.uk
Estée Lauder
www.esteelauder.co.uk
Green People
www.greenpeople.co.uk
Guerlain
www.guerlain.com
Ila
www.ila-spa.com
Illamasqua
www.illamasqua.com
Jane Iredale
www.JIProducts.co.uk
Jurlique
www.jurlique.co.uk
Kate Somerville
www.katesomerville.com
Kevyn Aucoin
www.kevynaucoin.com
Lancôme
www.lancome.co.uk
La Roche Posay
www.laroche-posay.co.uk
Laura Mercier
www.lauramercier.com
Lily's Nail Bar (NY)
15 E 21st Street, New York;
+1 (0) (212) 254 4118
Living Nature
www.naturisimo.com
Liz Earle
uk.lizearle.com
L'Oréal

www.loreal.co.uk
MAC
www.maccosmetics.co.uk
Make Up Forever
www.makeupforever.com
Nars
www.narscosmetics.co.uk
Nvey Eco
www.nveyeco.co.uk
Origins
www.origins.co.uk
OPI
www.opi.com
Prescriptives
www.prescriptives.co.uk
Proactiv
www.proactiv.co.uk
Ren
www.renskincare.com
Revlon
www.revlon.com
RMK
www.rmkrmk.com
Sarah Chapman
www.sarahchapman.net
Shu Uemura
www.spacenk.co.uk
Sisley
www.sisley-cosmetics.co.uk
Soap & Glory
www.soapandglorycosmetics.com
Spa NK
www.spacenk.co.uk/category/
spa.do
Strip Waxing Bar
112 Talbot Road, London W11
1JR; +44 (0)20 7727 2754
The Organic Pharmacy
www.theorganicpharmacy.com
There Must Be A Way
www.theremustbeabetterway.co.uk
Urban Retreat
www.urbanretreat.co.uk
Vanda Serrador at Urban Skin
www.urban-skin.com
Yon Ka
www.feelunique.com
Zelens
www.zelens.com

Acknowledgements

Make-up artists

Jemma Kidd

David Horne

Ciara O'Shea

Nicoline Divito

Pammy Cochrane

Marco Antonio

Tracey Quinn

Hair stylist

Davide Barbieri

Stylists

Alex Longmore

Elle Noble

Art director

Lawrence Morton

Commissioning editor/writer

Zia Mattocks

Photographer

Vikki Grant

Photographer's assistant

Emma Brown

Product photographs

Natasha Lewis

Models

Cecile (MOT)

Charlotte De Carle (FM)

Cherie (Nevs Models)

Gia (Zone Models)

Guadalupe (Nevs Models)

Hannah Phaisley (MOT)

Jasmine H (Union)

Juliana A (Nevs Models)

Karin P (Nevs Models)

Melanie Liburd (MOT)

Natalie Cox (Nevs Models)

Samantha Tea (FM)

Tanell (Union Models)

Tuan (Nevs Models)

Yulia (Zone)

With thanks to
Hannah Copestick, Mich Turner,
Maureen Thompson and
Mary Meikle.

Coordinator

Siobhan Conneely

With special thanks to David Horne, who contributed so much of his time and expertise to this project.

David is Director of Education at the Jemma Kidd Make Up School and has more than 20 years' experience as a creative catwalk make-up artist.

Thanks also to Grace Fodor, for all her invaluable support.

Grace is CEO of Jemma Kidd Make Up School.

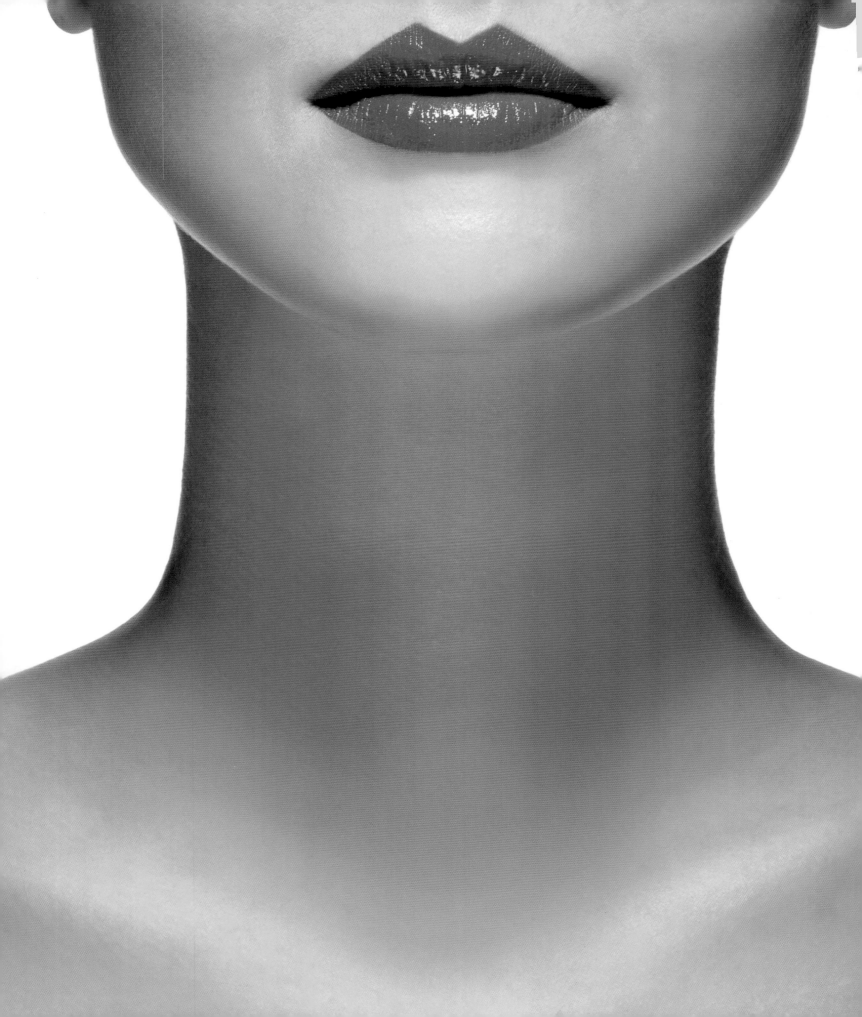

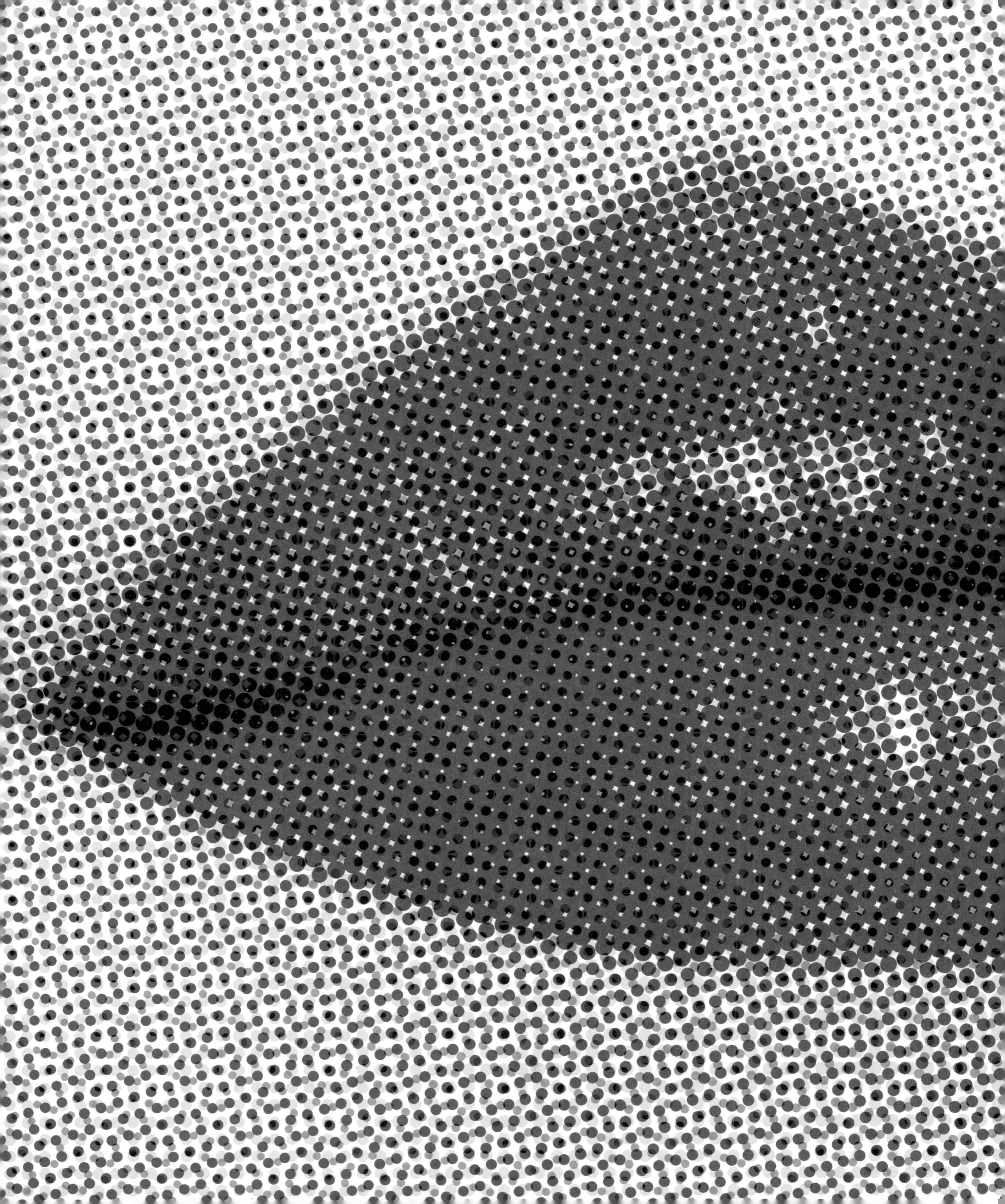